HEALED & READY TO FULFILL DESTINY

Bruised BUT NOT Broken

SHERMA ORIAKHI-MERSELINA

BRUISED BUT NOT BROKEN
Healed and Ready to Fulfill Destiny

Sherma Oriakhi-Merselina
sherma@kellyoriakhiministries.org

ISBN 978-1-949826-36-4
Printed in the USA.

Published by: EAGLES GLOBAL BOOKS | Frisco, Texas
In conjunction with the 2021 Eagles Authors Course
Cover & interior designed by DestinedToPublish.com

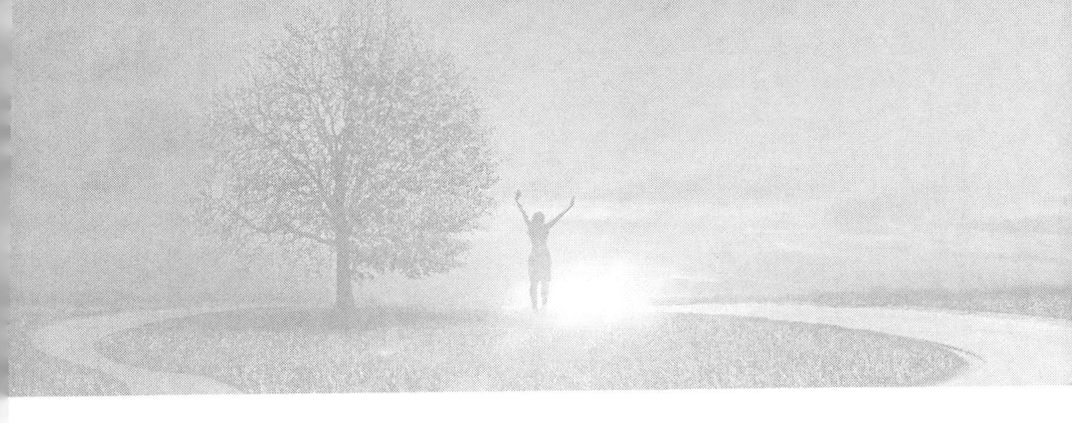

Dedication

This book is dedicated to all the vessels of God who have been called into the ministry, but who have been struggling to accept the calling or don't really understand it. To those who are walking into their calling but got stuck somewhere along the line and need to come back to the drawing board to rewrite the assignment given to them.

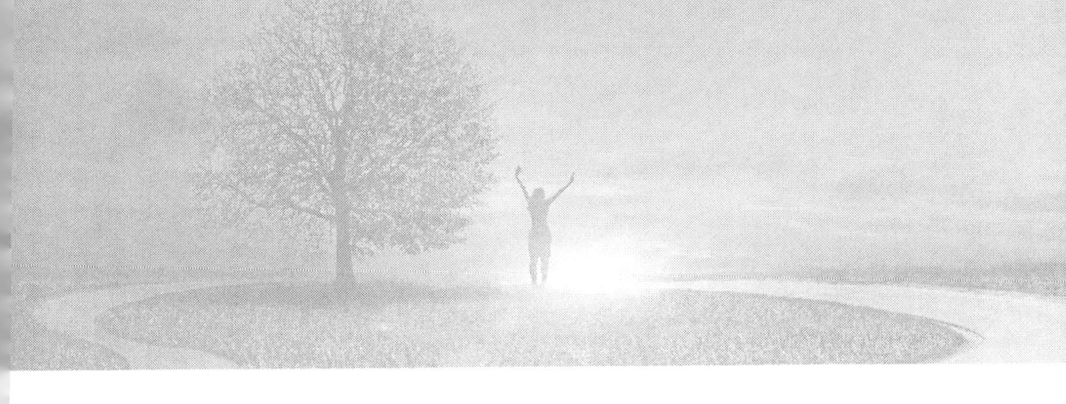

Foreword

This book will be a blessing to many.

Growing and changing is a must when we are serving God. We cannot stay the same as we first gave our lives to Him. When we say yes, sometimes we will experience growing pains. As we embrace His calling we also have to embrace the process, which is not always easy.

But once we surrender we will come out better. That's why I enjoyed reading your book and the examples you included.

I love how you are using your own life as a testimony. Love love LOVE the part where you are talking about your father and that God is now your heavenly AND earthly Father. You are complete!

I felt your heart where you write about the loss of your brother and family members. And how it affected you. I praise God for what He is doing in/through you.

Lech lecha! – Go forth!
Much love
Gaditcha Forbes Olijfveld

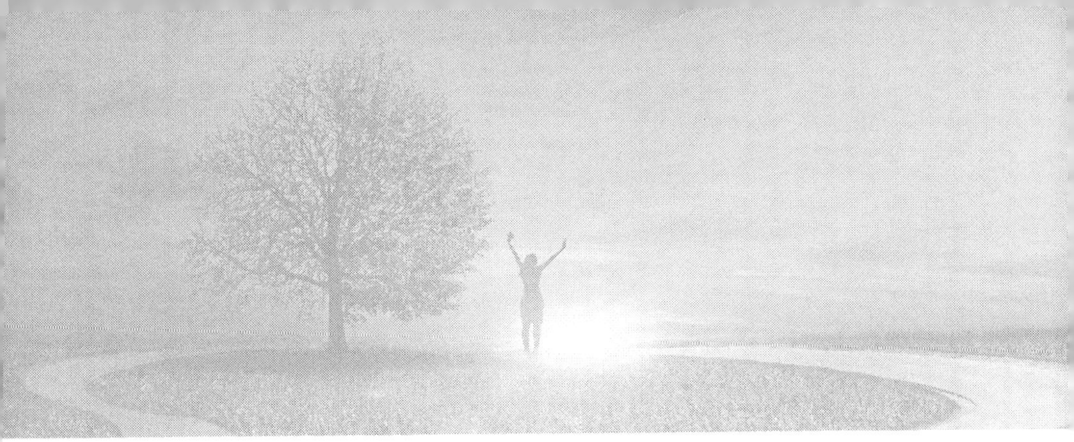

Acknowledgments

The Lord is my light and my salvation, so why should I be afraid? It is by God's grace that I stand and that I had the opportunity, courage and strength to write this book. Thank you, Father.

Apostle Kelly Oriakhi, my lovely husband. No doubt, you are my precious gift from God. Thank you for your support, love and patience. I love you very much, honey.

A big thanks to the teachers and coaches Marilyn Alexander, Deborah Anthony and Kara May from Eagles International Training Institute Authors Course. All those wisdom tools you give me helped me to finish this book. I am forever grateful.

To Apostle Gaditcha Forbes-Olijfveld, thanks for your willing heart to read my book and give me your honest feedback. I thank God for your life, family and ministry.

To my editor Erin, thanks for saying yes to this assignment. I am grateful.

Contents

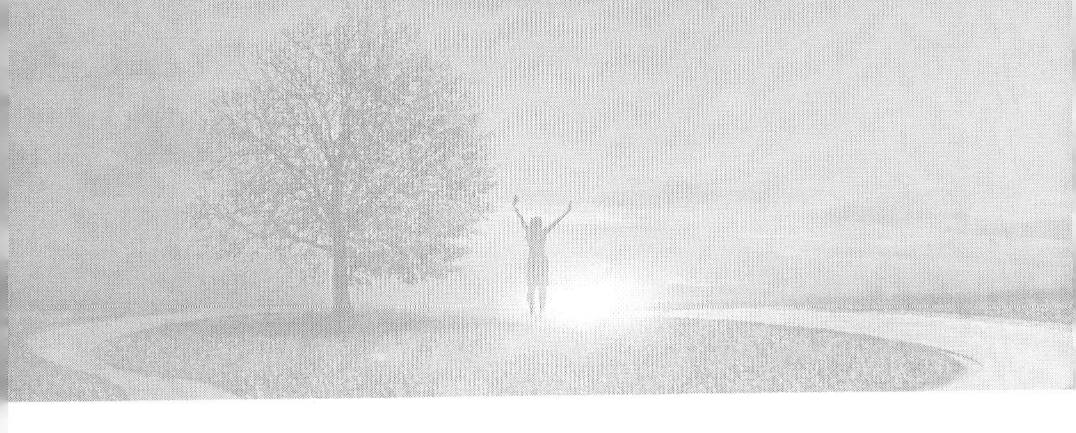

Introduction

This book is about your gift and calling by God to fulfill your assignment here on earth. It is he who called and formed men and give us an assignment here on earth. Work was the very first assignment God gave men. Right back in the garden of Eden that was the very first time that God gave men work. Answering to the assignment might never be easy.

You may go through many afflictions, struggles and pain before answering to the call. But once you say yes to the call, that is when you have signed up to a life journey with God holding your hand.

This book is written, led and inspired by the Spirit of God. I did some research on heart issues to get a deeper understanding about the heart, and I have spent some years following the patterns of certain ways people behave and relate with each other. That helped me understand how people behave (and how I behave) and how we deal with issues.

In this book, I talk about my own personal experience in dealing with matters and how I learned from the Word of God, with the guidance of the Holy Spirit, how to deal with them and answer to the call.

Chapter 1

To Be Called by God

The wedding banquet

"Jesus spoke to them again in parables, saying: 'The kingdom of heaven is like a king who prepared a wedding banquet for his son. He sent his servants to those who had been invited to the banquet to tell them to come, but they refused to come. Then he sent some more servants and said, "Tell those who have been invited that I have prepared my dinner: my oxen and fattened cattle have been slaughtered, and everything is ready. Come to the wedding banquet." But they paid no attention and went off– one to his field, another to his business. The rest seized his servants, ill-treated them and killed them. The king was enraged. He sent his army and destroyed those murderers and burned their city. Then he said to his servants, "The wedding banquet is ready, but those I invited did not deserve to come. So go to the street corners and invite to the banquet anyone you find." So the servants went out into the streets and gathered all the people they could find, the bad as well as the

good, and the wedding hall was filled with guests. But when the king came in to see the guests, he noticed a man there who was not wearing wedding clothes. He asked, "How did you get in here without wedding clothes, friend?" The man was speechless. Then the king told the attendants, "Tie him hand and foot, and throw him outside, into the darkness, where there will be weeping and gnashing of teeth." For many are invited, but few are chosen.'" (Matthew 22:1-14)

In the parable of the wedding banquet, we are taught that the kingdom of heaven is like a king who prepared a wedding banquet for his sons. He sends out an invitation for us to come to the wedding – an invitation to come and be part of something marvelous, a wonderful celebration. Let's try to understand that word "wedding." According to Thayer's Greek Lexicon, the Greek term is γάμος, γάμου, ὁ, which probably comes from a root meaning "to bind" or "to unite." Thus, a wedding is a covenant with two people joining together. You are no longer single. You are part of another person's life, and that person is part of your life. You are yoked to another person and have a covenant with that person. A covenant comes with responsibilities and commitments that need to be carried out. Another person is expecting something from you now that you have agreed to step into the covenant – meaning this covenant will affect your life. You will have to make some adjustments to live up to the agreement of this covenant.

When I gave my life to Christ for the second time in 2004, I made up my mind to go all the way. At that time, I didn't even know anything about covenants or what it meant to worship God. I just felt a kind of peace in my heart that I never had before, and it felt good. I did all that I thought was pleasing to God, all that I would like others to do for me, all that gave me peace. With the little understanding I had about serving God, I tried to give all my heart to serve him. I was not perfect at the beginning. There were times I would mix worldly behavior and thoughts. It was like, "Ooooh, wait – since I feel good doing this, this is what I should keep doing as a Christian." But I soon discovered that this was a wrong mindset. When you give your life to Jesus Christ, the old must die and make way for the new. Every old habit had to go. I couldn't keep living the same lifestyle and expect to have a relationship with God – I had to enter a covenant with God. I wasn't thinking about the word "covenant" then; my thoughts were, "I am serving God now, so I must read the Bible and stick to what the Word of God teaches me. Whatever is not in the Bible or in what I am getting from preaching or Bible studies, whatever is contrary to his Word, whatever makes me uneasy, I must not do it." I needed to make a change in my life.

At that time, I was living together with a man, and he had just bought a house for us to go and live in together. Even though I had my house and he had his house, we had decided to live together in one house unmarried. But after having an encounter with God, I had a change of heart. I felt the way I was living was not pleasing to God. I needed to change my lifestyle if I wanted to keep serving God, and

I just felt in my heart that living together unmarried was wrong. He bought the house, and in less than a month I told him, "I can't live together with you. I am serving God now." Serving God was not an option for him.

After this, my heart towards him started to change. I started seeing him like a loving brother or friend, and no longer a partner. It was like my covenant with him was over, and now I had entered a new covenant with God. I know God was at work there, because that feeling in my heart got only stronger and stronger. It was like wherever I went, I could hear God telling me, "You can't stay no longer in that relationship – you need to let go." I found peace in my heart, and one day I called him, and we talked in a friendly manner and agreed to end the relationship. I felt like billions of heavy burdens just fell off my shoulder. I had peace and rest. Shortly after breaking off the relationship, I met my husband, my destiny helper who I had to enter a marriage covenant with, because now I know better.

Whenever you make a covenant, your life is bound to change, because you are no longer on your own but part of another. For you to fit and become part of another, you must let go some of your customs and habits. This is also what God expects from us. When he calls us, he expects us to change and submit to the rules and commandments in his kingdom. He expects us to let go of the old lifestyle we lived when we were in the dark and step into his marvelous light, living a new lifestyle that is pleasing and acceptable to him.

God suddenly appeared to Abram when he was 99 years old and tried to cut a deal with him. To Abram, God said, *"Walk before me faithfully and be blameless. Then I will make my covenant between me you and will greatly increase your numbers"* (Genesis 17:1-2). To be part of a covenant with God and receive the blessings, there are rules and conditions attached to it. You can't enter a covenant with God and maintain your old lifestyle. Change must come. Some choose to change radically, removing everything old at once and embracing the new lifestyle right away, and some choose to change gradually.

When I gave my life to Christ for the first time in 1997, I chose to do good and follow what others was doing. With the little I knew, I tried to live a good Christian lifestyle. But in that same year, I left for Holland to pursue my studies, and I drifted away from the word of God. I didn't know much then, and I didn't have people to teach me the kingdom principles. The seed of the word of God that was planted in me didn't fall on good ground, and I fell back right into the world. It took me seven years to come back to the Lord. I accepted the Lord in my life and never looked back.

The call

You were born into this world in sin and therefore have no rights to eternal life. When a child is born, it has no knowledge of good and evil. It is when that child grows up and becomes aware of good and evil that he or she makes a decision. It is this decision you make that will determine your life path. You have been given free will by God to make a decision about who you want to serve, and your decision determines whether you will receive eternal life or not. Hence, when God calls us, it's because he wants us to have eternal life. You can only have eternal life when you accept Jesus Christ as your Lord and Savior and get baptized. By giving your life to Jesus Christ, you have gained free passage to eternal life. Jesus came as the Savior of the world.

A life without Jesus Christ is a life of sin, and the wages of that is eternal death. (Romans 6:23) But Jesus Christ came that we may be redeemed, saved from all sins and connected back to God. He nailed our sins on the cross and set us free from the death penalty. When God calls us, it's literally because he wants to have a relationship with us in his marvelous kingdom and save us from eternal death. This is why Christ needed to come, to restore that relationship with God. Christ was willing to die for us and deliver us from every sin to bring us back in contact with the Father. The blood of Jesus Christ made us righteous.

When I got saved for the first time in 1997, I didn't have much understanding about who Jesus is. All I knew was that Jesus is the name I need to call on as I pray, because it is in the Bible somewhere and others call on that name. I was just following what others were doing most of the time – I had no knowledge or understanding, and absolutely no wisdom. I said and did a lot of things in ignorance, because I thought that was how to serve God. But when I gave my life to Christ for the second time in 2004, my eyes and ears started opening. I became like a student at the feet of Jesus, just like Mary. I was hungry to know more about God. It was the only thing at that moment that was keeping me from death. I had made a choice to live, and I discovered that to live, I must hold on to Jesus, which meant I needed to know more about him. I had left my family behind, living in a foreign land for seven years, very depressed and even suicidal. I couldn't go back home, because I thought that would make me a failure, so I had nowhere else to go but to Jesus. I had to answer to that call.

The calling is for all who will accept it. It is by choice you will have to answer to the call of accepting Jesus Christ as your Lord and Redeemer. Jesus, with his death and resurrection, redeemed us and made us righteous.

However, not everyone will answer to this call. A rich man will never easily enter the kingdom of God, because money is his master, and most of the time, the wealthy don't see the need to accept Jesus as their Lord and Savior. Jesus explained this to his disciple when he said, *"It is easier for a camel to go through the eye of a needle than for a rich man to enter the kingdom of God"* (Matthew 19:24).

A rich man once told me: "Sherma, the greatest challenge that I have being rich is how to maintain that wealth, and most of the assets I have belong to investors." Basically, what he was saying is that most of his wealth doesn't even belong to him. He is just taking care of that money for others, making sure that the capital grows. Woe unto him if he goes bankrupt! His mind and focus daily is on how to keep all that money that belongs to others. As long as the money is growing and more investors are coming and he is happy, why would he want to accept Jesus Christ? The fact that accepting Jesus would mean he will have to pay tithes or be a blessing to the church with seeds and offering, that alone will be a big "NO."

In the story of the rich man in the Bible, he asked Jesus what he should do to enter the kingdom of God, and Jesus gave him two instructions. The first instruction was *"You must not murder. You must not commit adultery. You must not steal. You must not testify falsely. You must not cheat anyone. Honor your father and mother"* (Matthew 19:18-19). The man told Jesus he was already doing this. I can imagine seeing the smile on the man's face, feeling proud of himself. But then there was a second instruction Jesus gave him: *"Go and sell all your positions and give the money to the poor, and you will have treasure in heaven"* (Matthew 19:21). But this last instruction he couldn't follow; he was too wealthy to do that. Now we see here Jesus telling him what to do to enter heaven. There is an instruction and a blessing, and to receive the blessings, he must follow all the instructions. But this man was rich and had many possessions, and he was not ready to give up all the material things he had to receive eternal life. He wanted the blessing but was not ready to follow all the instructions. He was not ready to let go of the riches of this world and receive the heavenly riches.

Just like this rich man, it might be that you are well established with a good reputation, and Jesus is calling you into the ministry. Will you let go of all that you have and answer to the call? Will you trust God that he has a better and bigger plan for you? A plan much greater than what you already have?

Most of the time, you will accept the calling at a moment when you are facing challenges with your back against the wall. That is how I felt in 2004. Jesus was the only way out for me. It felt like there was no other way out for my misery. No way to run or hide, no one to talk to. That is when you will either cleave on to Jesus or sink deeper into the world of sin. You will be having many thoughts going through your head, both good and evil. You will hear voices speaking to you, both good and evil.

I remember when I was in Curaçao, not yet a believer in Christ, I used to have awful dreams and visions. I felt like I was not complete, like there was a gap in my life. I started studying with Jehovah's Witnesses for peace. Something to hold on to. Something that would give me hope for a better end. Many times, I would see myself in a dark hole, or even lying in a coffin in that dark hole. It was very scary back then, and I really didn't have the courage to speak to anybody about it. Who shall I tell? Who will believe or understand me? Back then, I didn't know God like I do now. I was trapped with the spirit of fear and very suicidal. Sometimes I would cry for no reason. I just felt like I needed to cry to fulfill my day. Studying with Jehovah's Witnesses helped for a while, but it sure didn't take away the fear and those scary dreams – as a matter of fact, it got even worse. But everything changed in 1997 when I gave my life to Christ for the first time, and then in 2004 when I rededicated my life. I can't even remember when those dreams and visions left. A shift of peace came upon me: I felt freedom, satisfaction and the will to live. And the more I studied the word of God and served the Lord, the more I realized I was not afraid of death. I learned that *"to live is Christ and to die is gain"* (Philippians 1:21).

Thank God I am in a better place now. Now that I have Jesus in my life, I don't have those dreams and visions anymore. I am now dealing with other challenges, because I am in the next phase of my life. Each phase comes with its own problems and challenges. But the more we know, it sets us free! Today, no matter what you are going through, just know there is freedom at the end of that tunnel, and Jesus is waiting to receive you with open arms.

Eventually, you will have to make a decision about which voice to listen to. It will be God or Satan – you can't serve both. Whatever decision you make will determine your future from that moment on. It will show in the way you talk, how you behave and the path you walk. Today, if you have not made up your mind yet to accept the calling, I pray in Jesus' name that you will.

Why does God call us?

1. To work for him

God created man in his own image and likeness and gave us work here on earth, according to Genesis 1:27-28. After creating all things on earth, God gave men work. He gave us power and dominion over all things on earth to cultivate and multiply them. It is our responsibility as human beings to work on earth using the authority given to us by God. The same authority and job description he gave to Jesus Christ in Isaiah 61:1-6 he gave to us.

God told Adam to name all that he saw in the garden. It was man that gave names to all things and animals here on earth, not God. God only gave names to a few people such as Jesus Christ. And when certain names need to be corrected, God steps in and corrects them. That is why you see that he changes some names of people in the Bible – their name must be in line with their destiny. God changed Abram into Abraham, a father of many nations, and Sarai into Sarah.

The book of Isaiah chapter 61 gives us a good example of our job description here on earth in the first six verses. This was the same job description God gave to Jesus.

---

a. Verse 1: To bring the Good News to the poor, comfort the brokenhearted, proclaim that captives will be released and prisoners will be freed

The Spirit of the Sovereign LORD is upon me,
for the LORD has anointed me
to ***bring good news to the poor****.*
He has sent me to ***comfort the brokenhearted***
and to proclaim that captives will be released
and prisoners will be freed.

---

b. Verse 2-3: To tell those who mourn that the time of the Lord's favor has come

He has sent me ***to tell those who mourn that the time of the LORD's favor has come****, and with it, the day of God's anger against their enemies.*

[3] To all who mourn in Israel,
he will give a crown of beauty for ashes,
a joyous blessing instead of mourning,
festive praise instead of despair.
In their righteousness, they will be like great oaks
that the LORD has planted for his own glory.

---

c. Verse 4: To rebuild the ancient ruins and revive them

[4] They will ***rebuild the ancient ruins****,*
repairing cities destroyed long ago.
They will ***revive them****,*
though they have been deserted for many generations.

---

d. Verse 5: To serve the flocks

[5] Foreigners will be your servants.
They will ***feed your flocks***
and ***plow your fields***
and ***tend your vineyards****.*

---

e. Verse 6: To be his priest

[6] You will ***be called priests of the LORD****,*
ministers of our God.
You will feed on the treasures of the nations
and boast in their riches.

2. To be part of his family

God told Moses, *"Have the people of Israel build me a holy sanctuary so I can live among them"* (Exodus 25:8). He created men and allowed them to build him a sanctuary because he wants a family. Physically, you have the same DNA as your earthly mother and father, and spiritually, you have God's DNA when you accept the calling. You become part of God's family. And family is usually close to each other – they look after and take care of each other. In that same manner, God wants to look after us and take care of us daily. He loves us and wants to protect us, because he is our Father. My husband always says, "God has no aunty or uncle, he is God the Almighty and can't be compared to nobody. He doesn't want to share his family with no other gods. He is God the Father, God the Son and God the Holy Spirit, the Three in

One." That is it. There is no other godly family. It is just the Three in One that wants to be our family and take care of us.

Being part of God's family means he wants to rest in us, to always be part of our lives and decision making. He put his Spirit, the Holy Spirit, in us to always be part of us if we will accept him. He wants us to always seek his face before taking any steps, to make him our number one source and to know that he loves us. He sent his only begotten Son to save us from eternal death, for whoever will accept him (John 3:16). He wants to inhabit in our praises (Psalm 22:3). God is a Spirit, and he wants us to worship him in spirit and truth (John 4:24). God wants us to serve him alone, and no other gods, because he is a jealous God (Exodus 34:14). He wants us to be holy. Our bodies are the temple of the Holy Spirit, who lives in us and was given to us by God – we do not belong to ourselves (Romans 12:1; 1 Corinthians 6:19).

For me, being part of God's family is the best thing ever. I was brought up without my earthly father. I remember for a long time, I used to cry on Father's Day. I would see everyone happy with their dads, and I had no dad to go to. I tried finding my earthly father for many years, and I even had a dream of his grave, but I kept coming up with nothing but false hope. A few years ago, I decided to let go and just make God my heavenly and earthly Father. I talk to God as I would speak to a person right in front of me, like a child speaking to her father. Many times I will sit on the floor and in a vision see him with my head on his lap, just comforting me and rubbing my head. Now, I have a spiritual father and mother, mentors and God as my heavenly and earthly Father. I am complete!

3. To separate us from the Gentiles

You are included among those Gentiles who have been called to belong to Jesus Christ. You were born in sin. But the day you accepted Jesus Christ and got baptized, you were no longer property of Satan but of God. You were brought by his blood (Ephesians 2:11-13). The blood of Jesus separates us from sin. Jesus nailed our sins on the cross and said, *"It is finished"* (John 19:30). You are no longer property of Satan but of God when you accept Jesus Christ as your Lord and Savior. You were plucked out of the darkness and grafted into his light. You are no longer part of the common society but part of God's heavenly kingdom. You are now an ambassador of Christ here on earth with a main assignment to win souls for God's kingdom, to take them out of the darkness and bring them into the light.

In 2020 the Holy Spirit revealed to me, through a broadcast I was a guest speaker on, what "the blood of Jesus" really means. About a week before the broadcast, God was already speaking to me about the power of the blood of Jesus. It was like I was in the school of the power of the blood of Jesus. But it was during the broadcast that my eyes were opened. As I was talking about the blood of Jesus, suddenly another speaker took over, and she said it was only recently that God gave her full understanding about the blood of Jesus – and this speaker is a well-known

Apostle. She said boldly, "I am not ashamed to say it, it is only recently I got full understanding what it really means to be covered under the blood of Jesus." Right that moment, it struck me: the God that spoke recently to her was the same God that spoke to me a week before the broadcast. It felt good. Then I realized, after all these years of being a believer in prayer and pleading the blood of Jesus, I now really understand that power the blood of Jesus has. I was shocked and embarrassed, but at the same time satisfied.

Now, as I say "the blood of Jesus," I say it with full conviction that there is power in it and that something must happen as I say it. Saints, it is never too late too learn. Being part of God's family is a lifetime of life lessons. Get ready to go to school every day until you leave earth. And never be too ashamed or embarrassed to say when you really get the wisdom on how to apply the mysteries of God's kingdom. You just might be helping someone get their deliverance. That Apostle really helped me that day to admit I had little understanding of how to apply the blood of Jesus. Maybe that's the reason some of my blessings are stuck, because I didn't truly know how to apply the blood of Jesus.

4. To fulfill the purpose he has called you to

"All things work together for good for those who love God, who are called according to his purpose" (Romans 8:28). God calls us to activate the gift and to fulfill the calling and purpose he has for us. The way God calls each person is different – the way God calls me will not be the same way he calls you. God

keeps calling the sinners. Some hear his voice and choose to ignore it, and some just can't hear the voice of God. But the day you say, "Lord, I don't need you, I have chosen Satan" (meaning you don't need God in your life), he leaves you alone. He will not force himself on you, and he will not keep knocking forever. Our God is merciful, gracious and gentle.

5. To know the truth and be set free

It has always been part of God's desires and plan for *"everyone to be saved and to come to the knowledge of the truth"* (1 Timothy 2:4). God is the truth, Satan is the father of lies. Walking with God is walking with the truth. The truth is revealed to us to save us from eternal destruction. Not walking in the truth will lead you to the path of hell – you will be walking in darkness. Each time I read God's Word about who I am and confess that Jesus is my Lord and Savior, I feel light and I'm blessed. I feel like I'm walking on water. I feel like I am the most blessed person in the world. I feel complete.

6. To make a new creation

"So if anyone is in Christ, there is a new creation: everything old has passed away; see, everything has become new! All this is from God, who reconciled us to himself through Christ, and has given us the ministry of reconciliation; that is, in Christ God was reconciling the world to himself, not counting their trespasses against them, and entrusting the message of reconciliation to us. So we are ambassadors for Christ, since God is making his appeal

through us; we entreat you on behalf of Christ, be reconciled to God." (2 Corinthians 5:17-20)

God wants to give us a new life in him. He wants us to put away all the old, the pain, the shame, the disappointments and struggles and embrace a new life. He will wipe away the old you and make you brand new in him, forgetting the past.

The above Bible verses really helped me in 2004 when I had just given my life to Christ for the second time. I kept telling myself, "I have a new life." I kept singing, "I am blessed to be a blessing. A new life, the old must go. I can't hold on to the old." The more I said it, I believed it and started practicing it. That is how I was able to end my relationship with my former partner when we were living together unmarried. That old life had to go and make way for the new.

The Kingdom of light and the kingdom of darkness

In the beginning, there was one kingdom: the kingdom of God, "The Light." But when Satan was cast down to earth because of sin, he took over earth. The earth became his domain, "Darkness." So now we have two kingdoms: the kingdom of God, the "heavenly kingdom," which is the light, and the kingdom of Satan, "the earth," which is darkness. Every human being was born on earth in sin, in the kingdom of Satan, but when you accept Jesus Christ as Lord and Savior and are baptized, you are saved and become part of God's kingdom. This means that if you are not part of God's kingdom, you are automatically part of the kingdom of Satan, since you can't serve both God and Satan at the same time. You can't serve God partially. The Prophet Isaiah prophesied about that light: *"The people who walked in darkness have seen a great light; those who dwelt in the land of the shadow of death, upon them a light has shined"* (Isaiah 9:2). And in Matthew, that prophecy was fulfilled with the coming of the Messiah: *"The people who sat in darkness have seen a great light, and upon those who sat in the region and shadow of death Light has dawned"* (Matthew 4:16).

Accepting that light is by choice. Joshua explained to the people that they have to make a choice about which god they will serve: *"And if it seem evil unto you to serve the LORD, choose you this day whom ye will serve; whether the gods which your fathers served that were on the other side of the flood, or the gods of the Amorites, in whose land ye dwell: but as for me and my house, we will serve the LORD"* (Joshua 24:15).

A covenant with God or Satan

Just as you can make a covenant with God, you can make a covenant with Satan, and each one is always by choice. When God calls us and we accept the calling, that means we have denounced every other god and accepted Jesus Christ as our Lord and Savior. We must then step into a covenant with God. It will show in our behavior, character and attitude. God gives us his only begotten Son Jesus Christ; whoever accepts him has eternal life (John 1:1-5). Accepting

Christ means walking in the light – a light that the darkness of Satan can't comprehend.

Just as God is seeking for our attention, Satan does the same. God calls us to pursue godly things and not to be carried away by the worldly things. Satan calls us to pursue worldly things and all that is dark and evil. Everything that will bring destruction, stealing, killing and no eternal life but damnation – that is Satan calling. That is the covenant Satan wants to make with you.

When Adam sinned, sin came upon man: "the Adamic nature." That Adamic nature makes men want to embrace the evil that makes you walk in darkness. The works in darkness are evil and always bring bad and evil results. They can never bring good fruits. The works in darkness are *"adultery, fornication, uncleanness, lewdness, idolatry, sorcery, hatred, contentions, jealousies, outbursts of wrath, selfish ambitions, dissensions, heresies, envy, murders, drunkenness, revelries,"* lies, covetousness, confusions, divisions and so much more (Galatians 5:19-21). But when you accept Jesus, these works can no longer be part of you. The just shall live by his own faith! Daily you must work out your salvation, keeping yourself away from darkness and remaining in the light. You are a son of the light and day, and not of the darkness and night.

Accepting Jesus Christ brings you into the light, the kingdom of God. Satan comes in and attacks the mind. He starts with stealing your joy and peace. He puts evil thoughts in your mind – thoughts that will make you uncomfortable and restless, thoughts that are contrary to the word of God, making you an emotional wreck full of anger, worry, confusion, fear and all sorts of deadly emotions. When you start believing his lies and accepting the way you are feeling as part of your normal lifestyle, he keeps knocking on your head until you are destroyed. The ministry of Satan has always been to steal, cheat and destroy (John 10:10). He steals your joy and peace; he cheats you from what belongs to you (such as your possessions) and he destroys everything that gives glory and honor to God. His aim is to destroy your life, home, family and the church: all the blessings and promises of God.

The year 2016 was such a horrible and painful year for me. But I knew I had to hold on to Jesus and declare that he is still on the throne. In that year, my only brother was brutally murdered by police officers as he was defending his girlfriend at a party. I remember at his burial, during the ceremony, I stood outside the whole time. I just didn't want to see him lying in that coffin, so I made sure I went to see him at the mortuary a few days before the burial. During the burial, as they were about to take the coffin away, I stopped them, walked in front and shouted at the top of my voice, "Jesus is still on the throne!" In that moment, a spirit of boldness came upon me and I just had to release those words. After, I started evangelizing everyone at the burial. To all his friends, I would shake their hands and tell them, "Jesus loves you." I would look them in the eyes and let them know there is still a chance for them. Every chance I got with his friends, all they could hear from my mouth is "Jesus loves you – get saved." I'm sure most of them were wondering, "Has she lost her mind? Your brother just got killed – how can you say Jesus loves you?" But it was the only reasonable thing I could think about to say to them.

After the death of my brother, three more family members passed away suddenly in December of that same year. One passed at the beginning of December, and two on the 28th. It was like I became numb for a while. I just didn't know if I had to cry, pray, read the Bible or worship. The doctors were even wondering if I was okay. I just kept telling them, "I am okay." They were like, "You just had such a heavy loss – how can you be okay?" I was fully aware of what was happening to me, but I also knew that God has a plan and it is not over until he says it is over. So, out of this whole awful situation that was going on, something good must come out. I was looking ahead to that something good.

What made me think like that was what my pastor in Amsterdam told me. God bless that pastor for revealing to me those words, which I will never forget. The day my brother passed, my pastors in Amsterdam came to my house to pay me a visit. They sat down with me as I was crying for about an hour, and then my pastor started talking. He said, "Sherma, cry as much as you want. Don't try to stop it. Let it roll." Another thing he said that I will never forget: "The memories of your brother are going to come like a movie. You will have a lot of flashbacks. Let them come, don't try to stop it. It will eventually become less and then stop." Just as he said, that is how my life went for the next five years. What made it even worse is that I kept having to go back to the scenario of how he was killed, because I had to discuss it with our lawyers. I had no choice. I had to learn how to turn that horrible movie and flashbacks into a reasonable case. I needed to be focused. I couldn't bury the story; I had to keep the movie and flashbacks rolling and learn to be strong.

Towards the end of January 2017, I realized the crying had stopped. I just couldn't cry anymore. It was like the grieving had entered into another face. I started to talk and had questions. I had questions for God. "Why so much pain, and all in one year? Is it because I disobeyed you, Lord? Is it because I sinned that all these people died?" All these people who passed were very close to my heart. I loved them very much, and it was all premature death. I already knew about the death of my brother because God had revealed it to me in a dream twice, but when it happened, it came as the greatest fear that fell upon me. I was like, "God, why? Me and my grandmother prayed and fasted about this two years ago to prevent his death. Couldn't you just listen to our prayer and cancel the premature death? Did it had to be so awful and shameful for my family?" And to make it even worse, for the next years, I had to deal with the legal case persecuting the officer who shot him.

Looking back, I was never angry with man for all those deaths that occur in our family in 2016. I was angry with

God. In November 2019, I had just been baptized in Israel at the Jordan River. As I stepped out of the water, I started getting deliverance, and I discovered I was angry with God for not saving my families in 2016. But in 2020, God started revealing to me why and how all these deaths happened. Doors were opened that needed to be shut. God started to show me how to shut those doors and adjust my lifestyle and prayer life for myself and family. It was like an open book. Suddenly, a peace came upon my family. In 2020 I remember calling my grandmother in Curaçao to tell her, "Granny, it is like there is a sudden peace that came upon the family. But we must keep on praying." She said she felt the same. That peace can only come from God. Satan can never give you that peace. Now I have a new covenant with God, written and sealed with the blood of Jesus. When you accept Jesus, get into a covenant with God. Sign a contract with God about why he should keep you alive. Make that covenant with God!

Acknowledge that you have been called by God

As we can read above, you have been invited by God to be part of his family. This invitation to align with the will of God is like an invitation to be part of a wedding. Therefore, the first step is to acknowledge the invitation with your "Yes." The next step is to get baptized. Accepting Jesus Christ as your Lord and Savior is not enough for you to enter into the kingdom of God: you must be baptized. There are many people that accept that Jesus Christ is their Lord and Savior but have never been baptized. Unless you are baptized, you can't enter the kingdom of God (John 3:5).

Jesus, God the Son, came down to earth in human flesh and gave us an example for how we should accept God's calling and what we should do to enter the kingdom of God. Jesus came and said, *"I have come down from heaven not to do my will but to do the will of him who sent me"* (John 6:38). In that same manner, you should acknowledge that you are called by God not to do your own will but to do the will of the Father who called you. And the Father has put his Spirit in you, the Holy Spirit, to guide. *"Those who are led by the Spirit of God are the sons of God"* (Romans 8:14).

Jesus got baptized by John the Baptist and was able to operate fully in his ministry. When John the Baptist tried to stop Jesus from getting baptized, he answered, *"It is proper for us to do this to fulfill all righteousness"* (Matthew 3:15). Likewise, it is proper for us to get baptized to fulfill all righteousness.

If Jesus the Son of God got baptized to fulfill his assignment, don't you think you also must get baptized to fulfill yours? Today, if you are not baptized, I pray in the name of Jesus that you will no longer delay it!

The cross to carry

The mind

"Then he said to them all: 'Whoever wants to be my disciple must

deny themselves and take up their cross daily and follow me. For whoever wants to save their life will lose it, but whoever loses their life for me will save it." (Luke 9:23-24)

"Therefore, since Christ suffered in his body, arm yourselves also with the same attitude, because whoever suffers in the body has finished with sin. As a result, they do not live the rest of their earthly lives for evil human desires, but rather for the will of God. For you have spent enough time in the past doing what pagans choose to do – living in debauchery, lust, drunkenness, orgies, carousing and detestable idolatry." (1 Peter 4:1-3)

Let's take a closer look at the above scriptures. To be a believer and follower of Christ means you must deny yourself and carry a lifetime cross. Nobody can carry your cross for you. Nobody can serve God on your behalf. They can pray to God on your behalf, but if you want to see hope turn into faith and come into manifestation, you must believe and serve God. Only you can do that. The people of the world have hope and not faith. It is only those who serve God who can have faith. And the more you practice that faith, the more it becomes trust! When you can trust in God, you can walk side by side with him or even walk before him, just like Abraham did. Abraham walked before God.

From the moment you accept Jesus as your Lord and Savior, you start denying yourself and carrying your cross: a cross that comes with daily pain and struggles to kill the flesh from evil desires. As long as you are carrying that cross, you are denying yourself, meaning killing your flesh and letting the Spirit of God lead you.

Accepting Christ means having a daily lifestyle of Christ first, and the rest is secondary. A daily life in Christ leads to the road of the narrow gate. *"Enter through the narrow gate"* (Matthew 7:13). Carrying your cross is all about renewing the mind and having a godly mindset daily – thinking, speaking and acting with a godly mindset. Not swearing, lying, cheating, killing, stealing, anger, worry, bitterness, gossip, sorrow and all the other things that lead to deadly emotions. NO! It is about you showing the nine fruits of the Spirit: *"love, joy, peace, forbearance, kindness, goodness, faithfulness, gentleness and self-control"* (Galatians 5:22-23). A mind full of love for Christ and for his people, not a mind full with hatred, bitterness and resentment. Jesus made it clear when he said that you must love, otherwise you can't be his disciple.

When I rededicated my life to Christ in 2004, I was so excited to serve God. Whatever I could lay my hands on to do in the church, I would do it. I became a jack of all trades and master of none in the church, laying my hands on anything I could get to do. I would be the first to come and the last person to leave the church building. I just wanted to serve God. I was not thinking about calling and discovering my purpose, because I just didn't know anything about that. I was just so naïve, thinking I just need to serve and love God and I will make it to heaven. I would study the Word and only attend meetings in my local church, because I was in my church seven days a week. My mind and concentration was not on discovering my calling or visiting other churches or conferences outside my church, because I just didn't know better.

All that changed in a split second when a guest speaker came from America and prophesied over my life. She spoke over my life, and it was like a whole new chapter of my life opened up. I started to get hungry to learn more about who Sherma is and what God really wants from me. Does God want me to work in all the departments of the church, or is there more to it? I had questions that needed answers. But like I said, she came into my life and prophesied, and then she left. God bless the prophetess that just comes to activate your calling and then abandons you – because that is how I felt, abandoned and stuck with myself. I started wondering, "Am I still going to make it to heaven? Who can help me with this new information about calling and assignment? Shall I talk to my pastor about my feelings?"

I was really miserable for some time. But then I noticed God starting to speak to me through my dreams and visions. I used to dream before, but after the activation, I started dreaming like crazy. I have books I wrote with some of my dreams going as far back as 2000. The dreams even made me more confused at a certain point, because I started having a lot of dreams and seeing them come to pass. I would even talk to people about some of my dreams. Some would say, "That is so true, thank you for sharing that dream with me." But others would look at me like "What are you talking about?" or I would get feedback like "Have you been talking to so-and-so about me?" Most of the dreams I was having were about families and people's sins. It was like I was invading in the privacy of couples. Their marriages, children and lifestyle were against the will of God, so they didn't like what I was telling them. Back then, I remember feeling like Prophet Jeremiah, the weeping prophet, because I used to weep daily. It was part of my lifestyle – every week weeping because of all I was seeing and hearing from God and from people treating me badly. Most people were not happy with what I was telling them, especially when they knew they were going through it but didn't want to hear it from me. It was like, "Who does Sister Sherma thinks she is, coming and talking to me about my private life?"

I remember even telling my pastor about my dreams. His answer was, "Sister Sherma, you are tired, you need to rest. Try to get some rest." Well, that even got me more confused, and even discouraged at a certain point. How on earth can he tell me I am tired and need to rest? It is because I am sleeping that I am having all these dreams. I was in my head thinking, "Pastor, I love you very much, but it is clear you don't understand me and can't help me. I need to find my help elsewhere." The challenge in finding my help was, how could I explain to people what I was going through without them telling me I am tired or looking funny at me like I'm crazy? I just decided to start looking around.

Another challenge I was facing is that I only attended my church meetings and didn't go to other meetings, because it was like my church was the only church in the world, and if I attended another church meeting outside my church, I would be a sinner. I was really poor in my thinking then. But thank God for the grace that came and delivered me from that. Once I discovered that I like to dance a lot during praise and worship, and that my movements were quite different from the regular church members, I decided to get closer to the dance team in the church. But I didn't join the dance team, because I was hurt and discouraged by what was going on. I started to feel like a stranger in my church. Therefore, I decided to observe what the dancers were doing, but I couldn't really flow with them. I then decided to join The Eagles Network (TEN) because I was told that was the school the dance leader was following. Following TEN made my relationship with my church even more awkward. It was like, "Who do you think you are, following a dance school outside? Do you think you are better than us?" They didn't use those words, but that is how I felt back then. There was just a gap between me and my church. I felt lonely and was always careful in sharing information with my church about what I was doing outside the church. That was really not a nice place to be.

Well, after I started following TEN, I decided to follow Eagles International Training Institute (EITI), and my situation only got worse. I found myself in a box with nowhere to run. And to make my case even worse, I met my husband around that time. Back then, he was Brother Kelly with a clear calling and vision written, who wanted to marry me and start a ministry. Then I became an alien in my church. If I was talking less after meeting my husband, I started talking in parables to avoid any misunderstanding in our awkward situation with my church. I realized I had no choice but to educate myself more about what was going on in my life, and I was not going to get that information inside my church. Some changes needed to be done. I started following classes outside my church – with the permission of my pastor, of course, but like I said, I was very brief with my information to avoid any awkward scenarios. As I was following EITI and attending conferences outside, I discovered there were classes I could follow that could teach me more about all these dreams and visions and what I was going through – EITI, "The Prophetic School," because I was flowing prophetic and needed to educate myself to understand how to operate in the prophetic. I just started following all the classes I could and attending as many conferences outside my church as I could, to learn more about operating in the prophetic. As I was doing that, I came across destiny helpers that were able to mentor me more on the prophetic. I had some wonderful men and women of God who helped me grow into the prophetic and the dance ministry.

One day, my phone rang, and it was that guest speaker who had come to my church about five years earlier and activated my calling. She said, "Sherma, how are you?" I will never forget that day. She spoke to me as if we were having daily contact. It was like she knew what to tell me. I was able to tell her what I was going through and how I was growing. From that day, I knew that this guest speaker is a mother to me. She speaks and puts order in my life; she speaks and changes happen in my life. She speaks and gives me homework to go and think about whether I am on the right track. She speaks and I can laugh and express myself; she speaks and I am encouraged to move forward, not looking at the past to keep me back. She speaks and there is always an "aha" (Rhema) moment. I learned to cherish and respect her. We don't talk every week or month, but whenever she talks to me, change takes place in my life and ministry. Today, after eleven years, she is still my spiritual mother. I have a better relationship with her and visit her home in America as much as I can.

If I had known what to do back then, my life lessons would have been different. I made a lot of mistakes that took years to correct. I spoke some evil words to people who didn't believe or understand me. At a certain point, I even became rebellious because I was just angry and lost. I started going to my church less often and avoiding certain people in my church. I stopped fulfilling my duties in the church, and I was very judgmental and critical. I remember telling the pastor, "This church is not a fivefold but some kind of threefold. There is only pastor, elders and pastoral team – where are the rest for the body of Christ to function in?" Maybe I was right, but I could have expressed myself better. Anger made me speak very harshly sometimes.

Who understands me and wants to really help me? That was my main question for a long time. But God sent me destiny helpers, and I was willing to listen to their advice and bring change in my life. I guess God wanted me to go through life lessons to bring out the better me. – that person who can now be a destiny helper to many. Unless I have gone through a situation myself, how can I understand a person and be able to help them? I thank God for the life lessons I went through in discovering my calling.

Changing lifestyle

When you give your life to Christ, you are no longer living under sin but under his grace. The day you gave your life to Christ, you became a new person, and the old person is gone. It is like pulling off an old and filthy garment and putting on a new garment (2 Corinthians 5:17). You are no longer condemned but free. Since you are now wearing a new garment, the old flesh – your former lifestyle or habits – must die. You are now a new and transformed person. Sin has no dominion over you, and the devil can no longer possess you. He can only oppress you sometimes when doors are open.

As a believer of Christ, you are now under God's covering and protection. You now have to rely and depend on God for everything. His word is the lamp to your feet and a light to your path (Psalm 119:105). And when things get rough and the old lifestyle is manifesting or wrong thoughts come to your mind, you must be strong enough to resist it. You will have to submit yourself to God and resist the devil, and he will fly from you.

Your body must suffer for the flesh to die, removing sin. As the flesh dies, the Spirit of God is at work in you. It is only when you are ready to pick up your cross that you can become a true believer in Christ. While you are going back and forth, you are still in the hands of Satan. But if this is you, I pray from today that you shall no longer go back and forth. You will stand firm in the Lord and pick up your cross daily.

Worship lifestyle

God wants you to worship him daily. Jesus offered up prayers and petitions with fervent cries and tears to the One who could save him from death, and he was heard because of his reverent submission (Hebrews 5:7). Jesus knew that only the Father could save him, guide him and lead him. He said that he did not do his own will but the will of the Father. So he would wake up early in the morning and separate himself from the rest and pray to the Father. Likewise, God the Father wants us to have that lifestyle with him, to seek him first daily. God wants to be daily number one in our lives. You must surrender totally to him, pouring out your heart, body, soul and spirit. Come to his feet and sit as a child at the feet of the Father. You must see him always as your Lord and Savior, and you can only do that after you have denounced any other belief or god. You can't serve two masters.

Your acceptance comes when you obey and follow his command; when you read and meditate daily on his Word;

when you pray in his name and no other name; when you give him your high praise (Hallelujah); when you boast about him; when you kneel before him; when your faith and trust is strong in him. When you are totally sold out for Jesus!

Jesus, God the Son, had a prayer lifestyle, offering prayers to God the Father day and night. All the prayers of the Son were heard. The Son had a relationship with the Father, just like we need to have a relationship with our Father daily. God wants to hear our voice daily. Jesus said, *"I will do whatever you ask in my name, so that the Father may be glorified in the Son. You may ask me for anything in my name, and I will do it"* (John 14:13-14). It is yours.

The Lord is holy and inhabits in the praises of Israel. When praises go up, blessings come down. Therefore, we must praise his holy name, that name that is above any other name. It is only through our prayers that our lives are secured. God wants to hear his word, the promises he has made over our lives. He wants us to perpetually involve him in every step we take in life – to ask for his approval, guidance, help, protection, comfort and supply.

Chapter 2

The Assignment for His Elected Ones

His elected ones

"Every high priest is selected from among the people and is appointed to represent the people in matters related to God, to offer gifts and sacrifices for sins. He is able to deal gently with those who are ignorant and are going astray, since he himself is subject to weakness. This is why he has to offer sacrifices for his own sins, as well as for the sins of the people. And no one takes this honour on himself, but he receives it when called by God, just as Aaron was." (Hebrews 5:1-4)

When God calls you into your ministry, accepting that God chose you to serve him must be seen as an honor, just as any other promotion you get at a regular job. Notice I mention a "honor" – that's because it is God that decides who he elevates, not man. It is what you do that will move God to elevate you. In the previous chapter, you read about what it means to be a believer in Christ. After you have said yes to Jesus Christ, the next step is to discover your ministry. Why are you here on earth? What is your purpose here? In other words, what is your ministry? Every believer in Christ has a ministry that needs to be discovered. What is your ministry, and what is the job description that goes with it?

Acknowledging the call to serve the Lord doesn't always mean that you know what your ministry and job description are, but as you become prepared for the ministry, you will discover it better. And if you already know deep down in your heart that your ministry is to be a servant in the fivefold ministry or to serve with your gifts and talents in the marketplace, in business, in politics or any other place, then you should embrace it. I will explain more about your spiritual gifts and talents in chapter 3.

When we look at the story of Jesus, we see that God came down to earth in the form of man, God the Son, to redeem us. He came into this world with a purpose and a clear assignment. According to Romans 5:8-9, through the shedding of his blood, we have been saved and redeemed from every sin. Right from the beginning of his ministry, Jesus knew that he had come to earth to save the unsaved, share the Good News from city to city to all who would accept it and die on the cross to redeem us. Fulfilling that assignment was a journey with many bumps on the road, just like you will go through many bumps on the road as you serve God. In chapter 4, I will talk more about these bumps, the hindrances that you may come across in fulfilling the call.

Understand the job description attached to the calling

Each person operating in their ministry receives a specific job description. Apostle Paul got the responsibility of preaching the gospel to the Gentiles, and Apostle Peter the responsibility of preaching to the Jews. The same God gave each of his elected ones a different assignment.

In God's kingdom, no two job descriptions are the same. Just as each person's ministry is different, so too is the job description different. That is where each person will have to discover how to operate in their ministry. As believers in Christ, we all have the job description of the Great Commission to win souls, but the rest of the job needs to be discovered. You discover it as you seek the face of God daily. God will speak and reveal to you, and man will confirm it. The confirmation usually comes through dreams, visions or a prophetic word. I will explain more about the confirmation in chapter 3.

Jesus understood his purpose here on earth. He understood the job according to the description that was given to him. He said he came to do the will of the Father, showing that he knew what he ought to do and how to do it: *"For I have come down from heaven, not to do My own will, but the will of Him who sent Me"* (John 6:38). Just like Jesus, we ought to do the will of the Father, not our own will, as he speaks and reveals to us.

The only way you can understand the job description for

the ministry is when you serve God. No matter how you are serving God, those life lessons will shape you and teach you to understand your ministry better. God called Saul, who later became Apostle Paul, a man set apart from birth as a chosen instrument to minister to the Gentiles and their kings and to the people of Israel, with clear instructions that he would suffer for the Lord's name.

Apostle Paul specified his assignment to the people, making it clear what he was called to do. He knew his ministry: he was appointed by God to be an Apostle. "*I am saying all this especially for you Gentiles. God has appointed me as the apostle to the Gentiles...*" (Romans 11:13). He had a relationship with the Father and the Holy Spirit. He allowed the Holy Spirit to be his teacher and guide as he was going from country to country to bring the Good News. He did his ministry right from the beginning through revelations from God. He was never part of the Apostles that Jesus taught; in everything he learned, he was led by the Spirit of God. In the book of Galatians 2:2, we read that he knew how to speak the gospel with those who were in leadership to make sure that the message he was bringing was from God.

Just like Apostle Paul, you must have a relationship with the Father and be led by the Spirit of God to fulfill the job description. Remember, the assignment was given by God to do according to his will. Therefore, you need to hear from God to know what to do. Many people are called into the ministry but never got the chance to birth out their calling and finish the race well. There are a number of reasons why this can happen:

1. *They were ignorant about their calling.* An ignorant person has no clue about his call. He is just in church knowing nothing about what God has called him to do or what he is supposed to do in life. And what you don't know, you can't have, even though God has reserved it for you: "*My people will be destroyed because they have no knowledge. You priests have refused to learn. So I will refuse to let you be priests to me*" (Hosea 4:6 ICB). The only way you can overcome ignorance is by becoming knowledgeable. Like the knowledge and understanding I am sharing with you in this book, I am talking about the knowledge and understanding of the will of God for your life, which can be accessed through a personal study of the Word of God, reading Christian books, or listening to the preaching and teachings of the ministers of God. In the book of Ephesians 4:11-12, we read how God gave the church the fivefold ministry for the equipping of the saints for the work of ministry, for the edifying of the body of Christ. Moreover, to train us according to his heart, God gave us shepherds who will feed us with knowledge and understanding (Jeremiah 3:15).

2. *They just don't know what to do and dare not ask for help.*

Many people mess up their calling because they refuse to study the Bible to get a better understanding of their calling. Just as they are not reading about their calling, they don't ask for help about it either. They would rather live a simple life and die without fulfilling the assignment.

3. *They are walking in doubts.* Walking in doubts about your calling and not getting the proper help can be very discouraging. You can easily get confused and feel lost. You will start doubting yourself and ask questions like "Am I really called?" You might even see yourself less. When people ask you who you are or where you come from, your first answer most likely will be "Ummmm..." instead of saying "I am Sherma Oriakhi-Merselina, a Prophet called by God right from the womb to bring the gospel to the nations through the dance ministry and verbal words." Next, you might say, "Well I think I am called to do this, blah blah blah," all with doubts and insecure and afraid of being judged. No confidence in God or in oneself.

4. *They were never recognized by their leaders to fulfill that calling.* When this happens, most of the time you are forced to develop your calling elsewhere. You know you are called, but you are not getting the help from

your pastor, so you will have to seek help outside your church. But the problem we most often see is that some people choose not to seek help outside their church, because they don't want to be seen as rebelling or they become uncomfortable with their pastor. The relationship with their pastor starts to get awkward, so they just decide not to seek help outside their church and just do whatever is available to do in their church. Finally, they start believing, "My pastor doesn't recognize my calling, so I am not called."

5. *They got caught up in the crowd and forgot about their calling*. Instead of seeking God to find out what their purpose in life is, they neglect it and follow the crowd. They just refuse to see that they might be different with an assignment that needs to be fulfilled.

6. *They rejected their calling and decided to do something else.* When the assignment gets hard and embarrassment, troubles, accusations, rejections, financial struggles, sickness and shame start knocking on their door, they just reject the calling. Their faith has diminished.

7. *They decided to embrace someone else's calling instead of their own.* When someone becomes comfortable following others who are doing well in their

assignment, it all seems like less stress and worries. But what they don't realize is that each person has their own cross to carry, and you can't hold a cross for another. God will never give you something you can't handle. Embracing someone else's calling and refusing your own is outside the will of God, and God will hold you accountable for that. He gave you time here on earth to do the job assigned to you, not to do someone else's job.

8. *Rejection is operating in their calling.* Working for God always comes with a price. It is a seed you are sowing in tears, pain, shame, rejection, contempt and persecution. But eventually, you will reap in joy. It is an assignment that life lessons will shape you in how to do the job better. If you are not focused on your assignment, every negativity will discourage you and drive you away from it.

9. *They started well, but somewhere along the line they got discouraged, bruised and broken, just like Moses.* They start doing whatever they can lay their hands on but have never been able to fulfill their specific calling. It is like they got lost somewhere along the way and were never able to pick up their true calling. The only way you can birth that calling is when you seek God

through fasting and prayer, study and meditate on the Word and seek help from those who are willing to help you birth out your true calling – your destiny helpers. Your true calling can be seen as the calling you were born to fulfill here on earth, just like Jesus was called to preach the gospel and die on the cross for us, and Apostle Paul was called to preach to the Gentiles, their kings and the Israelites.

What were you called for? Fill in the spaces below with your name and your calling.

I .... was called to ....

Understand "the Great Commission"

"Then Jesus came to them and said, 'All authority in heaven and on earth has been given to me. Therefore go and make disciples of all nations, baptising them in the name of the Father and of the Son and of the Holy Spirit, and teaching them to obey everything I have commanded you. And surely I am with you always, to the very end of the age.'" (Matthew 28:18-20)

But was the Great Commission only for the disciples following Jesus at that time? Certainly not! Jesus spoke to his disciples, giving them this command for what to do here on earth. But who are these disciples now? Let's take a look at the definition of a disciple. The Greek meaning of the word disciple is "mathētḗs," which HELPS Word-studies describes as "(from math-, the 'mental effort needed to think something through') – properly, a learner; a disciple, a follower of Christ who learns the doctrines of Scripture and the lifestyle they require; someone catechized with proper instruction from the Bible with its necessary follow-through (life-applications)." Therefore, you can't force a person to become a disciple. It is only when the person has made up his or her mind to become a follower that you can train them. A disciple must be a learner, ready to receive and follow what he or she has been taught by the teacher. You are a student with a teacher.

Jesus gave the command that we as believers must obey. There are eight things we need to understand from this Great Commission:

1. *It is a heavenly mandate given to us.* The reason why we came to earth is to win souls. – to depopulate hell and populate heaven.

2. *The Great Commission is our life purpose.* It is not negotiable, whether you want to do it or not, to receive your heavenly reward. If you do it, you will receive your heavenly reward, and if you don't, then no reward awaits you. "*Those who are wise will shine as bright as the sky, and those who lead many to righteousness will shine like the stars forever*". *(Daniel 12:3)*

3. You must accept Jesus Christ as your Lord and Savior

before witnessing to others. *"There is salvation in no one else! God has given no other name under heaven by which we must be saved"* (Acts 4:12).

4. *You must understand the power given to you.* You have that power to win souls! Jesus said: *"Very truly I tell you, whoever believes in me will do the works I have been doing, and they will do even greater things than these, because I am going to the Father"* (John 14:12).

5. *It is meant for all believers and followers of Christ.* Every believer in Christ ought to know how to speak about Jesus Christ and tell others to accept Jesus Christ as their Lord and Savior. You can't win souls for Christ if you can't tell them who Christ is.

6. *You are bringing the Good News to all, but not all will listen, and that shouldn't stop you from trying.*

7. *It is not just for those operating in the fivefold or church leaders.* Every believer in Christ must follow this command. You must win souls, you must teach/preach the Good News at all times. Those who are authorized by their church can also baptize.

8. *You don't need to get your Master's or PhD to bring the Good News.* All you need is to read and understand the Bible. When you understand the Bible, you can talk

to others about it. As you are talking, questions will be asked, and you will sometimes need answers from the Bible to explain yourself. As Jesus was walking about the earth, he was gathering the Apostles. Some were educated and some not, but he taught all of them how to bring the Good News. He was the Word, and it was the Word that taught the disciples about the Word. The best teacher ever! Winning souls is not about how highly educated you are, but about how much you know from the Bible.

9. *There is an assurance and promise that God is with us when we follow this command.* God wants us to do this and to be satisfied in what we are doing. We don't need to ask him – or anybody else – for permission to follow this command.

The Great Commission is meant for every believer and follower of Christ. It is a command and assignment we must fulfill here on earth to receive our heavenly reward. At the heavenly gate, when the first and second books are opened, all that you have done with your time here on earth will be revealed.

Confirming one's calling and election

Before man elevates you, God has already done that; man just confirms it when you say yes to the call. It is God that chooses his elected ones to serve him. As his elected one, you are called to serve God at all times without retirement. It is an assignment till death. You can't suddenly decide you are going on leave and not serving God anymore. As long as you are here on earth and are breathing, you will have to serve God anywhere and at any time as he instructs you.

Jonah tried running to Tarshish, but eventually he gave up and obeyed God. Just like Jonah, you might try to run from the calling – but God will keep on calling. He stops calling when you say, "God, leave me alone." Like I said previously, we serve a gentle God; he will not force the calling on you. It has to be your free will. He gave us a free will to make our own decisions, so he can only work with his elect ones when they say yes to the call. If you say no to the call, God will leave you alone, but then you are on your own.

Chapter 3

To Be Called by God into the Ministry

From the Old to the New Testament, God frequently called people to himself and to his work. He doesn't look at the outward but the inward. Neither does he look at race, gender, color or age. All God needs is a soul that will answer to the call. *"And those he predestined, he also called; those he called, he also justified; those he justified, he also glorified"* (Romans 8:30). Each person is chosen differently, in a different time and season. And it is God who decides when to make the call. It is just like a phone ringing. Will you then decide to pick the call and hear that voice telling you that you are chosen for a certain assignment on earth?

How do you know what your calling is?

Every person created by God is called. This means both believers and unbelievers are called to do something in life. But you must discover that calling. You may be called to work for God doing ministry or called to work outside the ministry. Not every believer is automatically called to do only ministry work. Maybe inside the church you can serve in your gifts and talents, and outside the church you are a police officer or designer. Maybe you like trading, traveling, buying and selling; in that case, it may be that you are called into the marketplace.

How do you know you are called into the ministry?

When you are called by God, the area you are called to operate in is typically what always draws your attention. – the things you know you feel comfortable with, the things that, no matter how hard you try to run away from them, they just keep coming back to you. Maybe you always see yourself teaching people, or you like to read and write and you have no problem reading many books, and everything that concerns teaching comes very easy to you without struggle. That is already a sign you may be called to be a Teacher. Or you may be very skillful in building, managing and giving instructions, and you love to help people grow; maybe you are called as an Apostle. Maybe you always have a lot of dreams and visions, interpret dreams, interpret tongues, can see and hear things about people's past, present and future – that is a sign that you may be called into the Office of the Prophet. Maybe you are called to operate in the field ministry instead of in the church. You still have to go weekly to the physical church building for service, but outside the four walls of the building, you are called to run a ministry. Your ministry outside the church is just an addition to the church to help build it. People will come to your ministry to be fed, trained and equipped, and then they go back to impart in their church.

Whatever you are called to be, you always display the signs of that calling. Sometimes you know at an early stage what you are called for, and sometimes you don't know, but God always sends help to guide you. You will just have to open your eyes and ears well and sharpen your discerning spirit. You don't want to be led in the wrong direction. When it is easy to discern what you are called for, the spiritual gifts start to operate, and as you continue to operate in the calling, you will grow and position yourself in that calling. But some people can't seem to figure out what they are called for, even when the spiritual gifts are manifesting. Usually, it takes a higher person in authority – a leader, pastor, prophet, etc. – to speak over their life or guide them to connect the dots and understand what they are called for.

But even when someone speaks over your life and tells you what you are called for, "You are called to be so-and-so," you must be able to relate with what the person is saying about you. You must already have known in your heart that this is what you are called for. All you needed was a little reassurance. But if you can't relate with what the person is saying and just decide to become what that person says you are, you will struggle to operate in that job description, because you were not called for that by God but by man. Before you start putting a title to your name or making future plans over your life, you must know for sure if you are called to operate in the fivefold, business, marketplace, politics or other job. A person can't impose that on you. Taking the right step on this matter is a decision between you and God. Therefore, before you start with any job, whether fivefold, ministry outside the church, business or marketplace, you must seek God to know for sure that you are on track.

What are the Spiritual Gifts?

Spiritual gifts are gifts given by the Holy Spirit to every believer of Christ. It is not a calling, it is a gift, something you can do because the Holy Spirit gave it to you. The spiritual gifts are only for believers, because unbelievers don't have the Holy Spirit operating in them. Spiritual gifts are not temporary, they are for life, and you can't give your gift to someone else. You can operate in this gift every day as many times as you desire, and you can operate in as many gifts as you want to. All you need to do is pray and ask the Father for it. You are given this gift to serve the body of Christ and not to serve only yourself. This gift is given to you to edify, comfort and exhort (the gift of Prophecy). These spiritual gifts will help you serve in your calling.

When you become born again in Christ, you are given spiritual gifts. These spiritual gifts and talents will help you to become the person God has ordained you to be. The unbeliever can't relate with the Holy Spirit and can't operate in spiritual gifts but only talents.

Spiritual Gifts

Romans 12:6–8	**1 Corinthians 12:7–10**	**1 Corinthians 12:28**	**Ephesians 4:11**
Having gifts that differ according to the grace given to us	To each is given the manifestation of the Spirit for the common good	And God has appointed in the church	And he gave the fivefold. The calling into the office of:
		Apostles	Apostles
Prophecy	Prophecy	Prophets	Prophets
			Evangelists
	Ability to distinguish between spirits		
Teaching	Word of wisdom and word of knowledge	Teachers	Pastors and Teachers
Exhorting			
	Working of miracles	Miracles	
	Gifts of healing	Gifts of healing	
Service		Helping	
Leading		Administrating	
	Various kinds of tongues	Various kinds of tongues	
	Interpretation of tongues		
Giving			
	Faith		
Mercy			

Source: Thomas Schreiner, https://www.thegospelcoalition.org/essay/the-gifts-of-the-spirit/

What are Talents?

The dictionary describes talent as a natural aptitude or skill that someone has. It is also a gift given to you by God, the ability to do something maybe others can't do. When Moses was building the tabernacle, God gave him skillful people to build it. Each person is talented or skillful in something; you just need to discover it and develop it. It might be in trading, inventing, building, creating or farming. You can only discover your talent by doing it, not by just watching.

Your skills or talents can diminish when you stop doing them. You might have to take classes to gain back the level you were before. Both believers and unbelievers have talents, but it is only believers that have spiritual gifts. Have you been able to discover your talents?

How does God call you for the job?

ABRAHAM

Abraham was called by God to leave his family and go into the wilderness because there was an assignment for him there. He left his home to travel to a place of promise (Genesis 12:1-9). Abraham left without any address to go to. All he needed to do was trust God. Sometimes God will give you an assignment that has many parts you have to work out. All he needs is for you to trust him with the first part of the assignment, and then he will reveal the second part to you. That's how he builds your faith and trust in him. After

Abraham had obeyed God for years, God tested him with his son Isaac. God asked him to sacrifice his son to see if Abraham would do it. Again, Abraham obeyed and went on a three-day journey with his son Isaac to sacrifice him. Even during the trip, when Isaac said to his father, "We have the fire and wood, but where is the sheep for the burnt offering?" Abraham didn't panic or get angry; all he said was "God will provide a sheep for the burnt offering, my son," and they kept on walking.

Abraham waited on God for years for this promised son, and now he had to go and sacrifice this son. But he didn't question God, he just obeyed and trusted God, and for that he was able to pass the test. He was a man ready and up to the task given by God.

DAVID

When God asked Samuel to go and anoint David, he didn't give him a physical description of what the person would look like. All God needed was Samuel's obedience to go and do what he was instructed. *"But the Lord said to Samuel, 'Don't judge by his appearance or height, for I have rejected him. The Lord doesn't see things the way you see them. People judge by outward appearance, but the Lord looks at the heart'"* (1 Samuel 16:7).

Maybe you've been struggling with your appearance and seeing yourself as unfit to be a servant of God. You might be thinking, "I am a midget, an albino, deaf, blind, stuttering or lame," or whatever dysfunction you are dealing with on your body. "I can't serve God. People will not take me seriously." But the question that needs to be answered is, don't you think that God already knows your appearance and knows that you are the perfect person for the job? Physical appearance has never been a precondition for the call. God can use anybody or anything to do the job.

SAMUEL

In 1 Samuel 3:1-10, we see God calling Samuel, a little boy of twelve years old, to come and serve him. *"Now in those days messages from the Lord were very rare, and visions were quite uncommon"* (1 Samuel 3:1) – Samuel was called to do something very rare. Just like he did with Samuel, God can also call you to do something very rare.

Samuel's first time hearing God speak to him was about his leader, the priest Eli. God said to Samuel about Eli, *"I told him that I would judge his family forever because of the sin he knew about; his sons blasphemed God, and he failed to restrain them"* (1 Samuel 3:13). Can you imagine if it was you hearing this from God about your leader, and your leader forces you to tell him what God said just as you are about to start with your ministry? Would you have done it? The next day when Samuel woke up, he was afraid to talk to Eli, but he spoke to him and told him all that God said.

When God called Samuel, he thought it was a human been calling him. He thought it was Eli calling him. Because he went to Eli three times and asked did you call me. Just as he did with Samuel, God calls us and speaks to us with human voice – a voice that may sound familiar to you, a voice that will make you comfortable and want to listen to the instructions you are getting. Samuel was able to hear and understand when God was speaking to him, because he told Eli all that God told him.

When Samuel was called, he was just a lad. He didn't know anything about hearing the voice of God. He needed to be mentored and trained to learn to hear from God. There are many who have been called in their youth and needed to be mentored well before stepping into the call. No matter how anointed you are and how well you hear God's voice, you will still need to be mentored. Samuel was under the mentorship of Eli and was taught all he needed to know to walk in his calling as a Prophet. He was so well mentored that he became the national Prophet in a time and season where there were no Prophets. Anointing will make you start the ministry, but it is good character that will make you keep walking in your ministry. This principle of mentorship and training has not changed. Everybody needs to be mentored and trained to finish the assignment on earth well. Without training no discipline, without discipline no character, without character no prudence and without prudence no crown of glory.

KING SAUL

"There was a man of Benjamin whose name was Kish the son of Abiel, the son of Zeror, the son of Bechorath, the son of Aphiah, a Benjamite, a mighty man of power. And he had a choice and handsome son whose name was Saul. There was not a more

handsome person than he among the children of Israel. From his shoulders upward he was taller than any of the people." (1 Samuel 9:1-2)

"And Saul answered and said, 'Am I not a Benjamite, of the smallest of the tribes of Israel, and my family the least of all the families of the tribe of Benjamin? Why then do you speak like this to me?'" (1 Samuel 9:21)

Saul didn't expect God to call someone like him from the smallest tribe in Israel. Also, his family was not popular – in other words, they were "nobody" in the eyes of men. Nowadays, you are classified as popular when you have many followers and likes on social media. So, we could say that they didn't have many likes or followers on social media. Even Mr. Google might not even bring them up as first in the search results, because they are just not popular. Yet God called Saul, a member of this family, because his description was just fit for the job. The Bible records that the Israelites wanted a king. This was against the will of God, because God wanted to be the King over his people and not to have a human being as king. But God chose to harken to the voice of the people, and he gave them a man as king.

Saints, it is God that decides who is fit for each job description in his kingdom. You don't get to decide whether you are called to operate in the business market or ministry. It is God that decides what you are called for, and it is your job to discover it. *"The secret things belong to the LORD our God, but those things which are revealed belong to us and to our children forever, that we may do all the words of this law* (Deuteronomy 29:29). *"It is the glory of God to conceal a matter, but the glory of kings is to search out a matter"* (Proverbs 25:2).

GIDEON

Gideon saw himself as small and not capable of doing the job. He started bringing up all manner of excuses for why he could not do the job. But God already had a plan, and Gideon was the right man for the job. *"'But Lord,' Gideon replied, 'how can I rescue Israel? My clan is the weakest in the whole tribe of Manasseh, and I am the least in my entire family!'"* (Judges 6:15).

QUEEN ESTHER

Esther was a woman born with a great destiny and assignment to save her people from total destruction. But to secure that, she needed to understand that she was born for that assignment and take the job description seriously. God made sure she married the king to give her the power, courage and authority to speak to the king. And when it was time for her to speak, she fasted and prayed and made up her mind, *"If I perish, I perish"* (Esther 4:16), because the job needed to be done.

Women are called into any field just as men are. Like I said, God knows the exact job description for each person; all that is needed is for the person to answer to the call. There are certain jobs in certain seasons that need to be done by a woman, and other times, it can only be done by a man. God knows exactly who is needed in each season for the job and makes the call. But the question is, are you willing to answer to the call? Do you see yourself called by God for the job? Can you trust God in the job description? Remember, he said he will be with you.

APOSTLE PAUL

"As he journeyed he came near Damascus, and suddenly a light shone around him from heaven. Then he fell to the ground, and heard a voice saying to him, 'Saul, Saul, why are you persecuting Me?' And he said, 'Who are You, Lord?' Then the Lord said, 'I am Jesus, whom you are persecuting. It is hard for you to kick against the goads.' So he, trembling and astonished, said, 'Lord, what do You want me to do?' Then the Lord said to him, 'Arise and go into the city, and you will be told what you must do.'" (Acts 9:3-6)

Paul was a top persecutor of the Lord's people. Nowadays, we would call him a criminal, discriminator or maybe even terrorist to the Christians. He was on his way to Damascus, planning to execute his evil plans to persecute all the Christ-believers. To make it even worse, he was well educated and he was a man of influence. I want to believe getting to the top boss to work out his evil plans was very easy. He was deep in sin – and yet that was the man God called to write one third of the New Testament led by the Spirit of God. Yes, God calls even the biggest sinners to work for him. I believe it is even better when he calls the biggest criminals in the world and they answer to the call fast – we should rejoice more, as it makes the world more safe and enjoyable.

How did God call you? Write your name in the space below and describe it.

Chapter 4

Hindrance for Answering to the Call

Answering the calling is one thing; walking in the calling is another. After answering the calling, you have signed up to become part of the army of the Lord. And an army fights war on the battlefield, so you can't expect to say yes to God and have a peaceful life without any wrestling. *"We wrestle not against flesh and blood, but against principalities, against powers, against the rulers of the darkness of this world, against spiritual wickedness in high places"* (Ephesians 6:12). In the fight we are fighting, we can't pick up a gun and shoot the devil. The devil will just look at you, laugh and send even more enmity because of your ignorance. The fight you will fight is first spiritual, then physical. I always say being a Christian means 90% spirit and 10% physical battle. Most wars you will have to fight are spiritual. Therefore, the earlier you understand that, the better for you. Otherwise, you will suffer for years if you don't know what you are dealing with and how to battle it.

Get ready to battle for your breakthrough

First, you need to understand that this war you will have to battle is first in the spirit, and it manifests later in the flesh. It is evil spirits coming against you, trying to stop you from answering to the call. Satan and his agents will come against you in all sorts of manners just to stop you from fulfilling the calling. Satan doesn't like it when Saints have been promoted to a higher rank, so he will try to frustrate you. You will have to open your eyes and ears well, and speak and act in wisdom and guard your heart. In my book *Guard Your Heart,* I wrote about the things you need to do to guard your heart from the devices of the enemy.

The war you will have to battle can come from your home, family, friends, business partners, colleagues, customers, clients, your health, your finances, church members, your spiritual sons and daughters, spiritual parents, biological parents, brothers and sisters anywhere. But it is during those battles that your life will be shaped and made ready for the assignment given to you by God. These battles, I call them "life lessons." Each battle you go through is a process, and each process goes in phases and seasons. And whatever you say, believe or do, you become, so if you believe this battle, you have already overcome it, and if you walk as a victorious person, you will indeed win the battle. But if you believe the opposite and present yourself in that manner, you have already lost the battle. Each life lesson must bring out a promise, prophesy or product. I call it the 3-P. As long as you don't see the outcome of your promise, prophesy or product being fulfilled, you are still in that process of life lessons.

Think of plants that go through two or four seasons yearly and always blossom. The plant knows there is a season when it might look dead outwardly – brown, dry, no leaves – but it is not dead. It is just preparing the inward for the blossom season. The same goes for human beings in knowing what season you are in. There is the season when you may look dry, worried, confused and exhausted; you may be going through a lot of shameful things, with arrows of false accusations coming at you from left and right, discouragement, less faith, financial dryness, family suddenly misbehaving, all sort of attacks. But then comes that season when you will start to read and hear more of the word of God and be able to fast and pray; you will start walking with destiny helpers and begin to gain strength. Then comes the season where you can hear the voice of God very clearly and start seeing the light, the end of your struggles and where you can start preparing for your breakthrough. Know which season you are in.

After his baptism, Jesus had to go through that process too before he could start his ministry. He had just been baptized, and he was led into the wilderness to be tempted by Satan. Satan was trying to stop him from fulfilling the assignment. But Jesus was wise enough to see and understand this. Jesus told Satan three times, "It is written," referring to the Word of God, and the third time he commanded him, "Away from me, Satan!" (Matthew 4:10). Jesus resisted Satan, who flew away from him. Jesus knew the Word of God, and even Satan himself knew it and was using it to manipulate Jesus. But Jesus knew you can't put God to the test. You can't manipulate God using his own words against him.

Saints, just as Jesus was able to resist Satan, you will have to do the same to answer to the call. Submit yourself to God, resist the enemy, tell Satan to get lost. He is under your feet, and he will flee from you (James 4:7).

The process of each battle you go through may not be sweet. But when you hold on to Jesus, he will make you stronger and wiser. He will wipe your tears.

What are some of the hindrances you will go through when you are called into your ministry?

1. Ignorance

Out of ignorance and a lack of understanding, you don't answer to the calling at first. You don't even understand it. You are just doing as you are told; you have not been able to discover your calling or vision. You are in such ignorance that you become jack of all trades and master of none. It is good to work, because God hates idleness and encourages us not to be idle. At a certain time in life, you most move from that level of whatever you can lay your hands on to your specific calling into your ministry. That is when your knowledge and your relationship with God are growing.

Gradually, you start to understand God's calling upon your life. From a state of ignorance, you graduate to a specific calling. Then you must move from doing general things into doing the things God has called you to do.

Jacob worked for Laban for years. He did all that he could do for Laban. Jacob spoke to his wives, Leah and Rachel, reminding them of how Laban, their father, had deceived him and changed his wages ten times. Yet God had been with him, and whenever Laban had changed his wages, God had ensured that Jacob would be blessed in spite of his father-in-law's underhanded schemes. But at a certain point, Jacob said, "I can't continue like this. I need to do something for my own household." And he was willing to work for it. This is when Jacob moved into the specific calling upon his life. Jacob was not operating in the fivefold, but he was an inventor and businessman.

Just like Jacob, each person at a certain point must discover their purpose in life and do what they need to do to achieve their goals. When you are doing whatever you can lay your hands on, you are just gathering experience for your next step in life. But then you need to know for what purpose you are gathering all these experiences. There must be a reason. That is when you refuse to be ignorant. After you have gathered all the experience you can, just like Jacob, you must move to the next step in life: your own household, your own calling. One day, a mentee called me, and she said, "Prophetess, I am tired that every month I have to study twice as hard to submit my assignment. It is very exhausting for me. What shall I do?" Right that moment, the word of wisdom came to me. "First of all, every month you have to study hard, but your score remains 100%. God is just preparing you for your next phase to become a good teacher in what you are studying. By the time you are done, you will be able to master the course with no doubt in your heart how to go about your ministry." She was just amazed at my answer, because she didn't see it in that manner.

Once you have discovered your calling and are willing to step into that phase in life, it brings fulfillment that money can't buy. Until you move into your specific calling in life, you don't find fulfillment. When you move into the specific calling upon your life, money, favor, honor, breakthrough and growth don't come right away. They come later. But when you develop a prayer lifestyle, asking God what you want to achieve or see in your ministry, you start seeing your blessings. Just have patience and trust in God that it will come, because they are all part of your blessings. The first thing you get when you are doing what God has called you to do is fulfillment on the inside. Even when you have no food or money, you have self-fulfillment. Nothing is greater than that. May you move from ignorance to assurance in Jesus' name.

2. Fear

"For God hath not given us the spirit of fear, but of power, and of love, and of a sound mind." (2 Timothy 1:7)

Fear is just false evidence appearing real. As believers, we shouldn't be afraid. In my book *Guard Your Heart*, you can read a lot more on fear. There are many reasons why fear might keep someone from answering to the call. I will start with myself.

When God was calling me into the Prophetic ministry, I thought, "I can't do this, because I am afraid of making mistakes. What if I give people prophecies that are not true? Will I end up in hell?" Very dreadful thoughts. I decided to get help from my mentors and spiritual parents and schools to understand my ministry. It took me about ten years to understand my calling, and I am still learning every day. It seems like when I didn't know I had been called to be a Prophet, life was much easier. I would speak with so much conviction, not even thinking of the consequences. And all the dreams I would have each day were nice, especially when I would see them come true. I felt special that I could have all those dreams and speak about past, present and future. I know things even before they happen. But when I got the full understanding that I would be held accountable in heaven for all that I do on earth, I became afraid and tried to run away from the Prophetic. I started talking with doubts, using words like "I am not sure, but I think this is what I am hearing." You know that kind of feeling like you don't want to be blamed for mistakes. I had to learn when and how to speak, how to have a personal relationship with God and how to listen to him and see what he wants me to see. I had to learn to understand that not everybody can do what I do. Not everybody is a Prophet, and each Prophet operates differently as you are led by the Spirit of God.

Fear will keep knocking on your door when you are not sure about your calling or how to operate in it. That is why you will need to get help. No man has ever been able to operate in their calling without help. You will need help, and God always sends help. But even when help comes, you will have to take a leap of faith and acknowledge who you are. Remember that the calling and gift upon your life is irrevocable. You can't run away from it. It is inside of you.

The calling might be irrevocable, but you are not indispensable. You can be replaced by God at any time. When Saul messed up, God replaced him with David. You must take the calling upon your life seriously and work out according to God's plan. You must always be in line with God to operate in your calling. All you need to do is activate it and allow the Spirit of God and destiny helpers to guide you into the calling. Remember, God said he will be with you, so you don't need to be afraid. He gave you the calling and the gift, and he will take care of you. Even when your mother and father forsake you, he will take care of you. Allow God to use you, and don't be afraid.

3. Rejection

Rejection is a spirit that comes with the main goal of destroying everything about you: your life, family, work, ministry, business, career, relationships and church-going. Most of the time, this spirit comes in at an early age. Maybe by birth you were rejected. Or even in your mother's womb, maybe she wanted to abort you, so she denied she was pregnant and didn't protect the pregnancy. You can even deal with the spirit as an adult churchgoer. That seed of rejection starts growing in you and creates a wall of your own world: a world where it must be about you and only you, because you believe the world always wants to ill-treat you. You try to find others who are vulnerable and going through similar situations, and they become your friends. You have the need to want to protect only those inside your world; the rest is not relevant. Your focus most of the time is "me, myself and I." You will do whatever you can to get what you want. Most of the time, you don't think of the consequences. Dealing with the spirit of rejection makes you very selfish and self-righteous. It makes you always want to create pity parties. You can easily try to manipulate and control people or situations.

I remember when I was dealing with this spirit, I was very controlling and dominant. If I didn't get what I wanted, it made me very angry and I would easily separate myself. Now I am free from this spirit, and whenever it tries to knock on my door, I just rebuke it in Jesus' name. I ask God to break me and mold me, to show me daily his ways. That is why I love when people give me feedback, and I take time to evaluate myself. I learned to be honest with myself. Am I still on track? Did I miss it somewhere along the line? Where in my life needs correction because I allowed this spirit of rejection to enter? I learned to be a good observer and listener, to ask questions and dare to say I am sorry whenever I am wrong. Another thing I learned is to stop crucifying myself for my past mistakes or my denials. I can't erase them, but I can make my now better by the wisdom of God and be led by the Holy Spirit.

I remember answering my calling and dealing with this spirit – it made me very controlling. I wanted people to stop rejecting what the Lord was telling me. I needed them to embrace the prophetic word. I soon realized I had been looking for confirmation of the word that was coming out my mouth. It was like I wanted to prove that what I said is true, that I wasn't lying. When I discovered what I was doing, I felt so ashamed of myself. Before I realized, it was like I was trying to take the glory that belongs to God. Now I drop the word whether you want to take it or not – that is between you and God. My mind and focus is no longer in seeking to find out if the prophecy has come into fulfillment. Now, people will come to me and say, "Prophetess that word you gave me back then, it came to pass," and I will respond, "Please remind me what I told you." I just can't remember the word most of the time. My mind is just no longer there unless God gives me an assignment to pray through that prophecy. I will keep watch till I see it come into fulfillment. I usually pray early in the morning from 3:00 a.m. for people to start their ministry; after that, another prayer point will come, and I will keep on doing that till I no longer have it in my heart to pray.

For years I have been praying for friends, family and even my enemies for change and blessings in their lives. Nothing gives me more joy than to see the change in their lives. Especially my enemies – I just pray and pray, and God will just make a way and bring healing. He might use a third person to talk to us, or he will just start opening up our eyes to see the truth and bring healing and restoration in that situation. I remember for a long time I had to pray for some leaders who were disparaging me and my ministry. They just looked down on me and my ministry, but at 3:00 a.m. I would be praying for their ministry, home and children for God to bless them and make them great. Doing that, I felt good; I felt like being a faithful and humble servant of the Lord. I chose to focus not on the way they treated me but on the bigger picture: the part where the problem can be discussed, forgiveness comes in and the healing process can start. I chose to think and act positively and wait on God to take over the battle.

4. Low Self-Esteem

This spirit comes in and makes you feel useless. Usually, when you are dealing with the spirit of rejection, you have low self-esteem. Low self-esteem makes you think you can't make it. You never see yourself as a winner but as a loser. You will encourage others but can never encourage yourself. Most of the time, you live in denial. I remember trying to help quite a few people dealing with this spirit, and at a certain point, I started to wonder, "Does this person have love?" I soon discovered the answer is no. A person dealing with low self-esteem doesn't really know what love is. They select the ones they want to love. When you give them positive feedback, bless them with nice things or spoil them, they love you and will accept you. But when you start correcting them, they write you off very fast. They mainly pretend all is well, but in their hearts it is not well. They will not always speak the truth to you. They will say "A," but meanwhile they are thinking "B." They will accumulate, and when they start boiling, they will spill it out very negatively.

When you are dealing with this spirit, it makes it very difficult to see that when you are doing God's work, it is not about you but about God. When people hurt you after you have just preached the word of God to them with a sincere heart, you want to take it personally. Please remember that as you preach the gospel, some will hate you and some will love you for Christ's sake. Whatever your calling may be, just know that there will always be some who will like you and some who will not like you. You will have to look beyond that and focus on your main goal. What do you want to achieve?

5. Insecurity

Like with low self-esteem, people dealing with insecurity are good at pretending. They would rather pretend and hide the truth. Being insecure will hinder you from obeying God. You will not be able to obey God's voice, because your focus and attention is on "What will people say or think of me?" Remember, it is not about you but about God. I remember when I was not sure if I was called as a Prophet, I used to say "I think and feel in my heart such-and-such." I would not dare to say "Thus says the Lord." I would start to negotiate with God. "God if it is really you speaking, give me a few confirmations." Before I knew it, God would use another person to deliver his message in the same way he gave it to me. I really felt stupid each time that would happen. Now, I have learned to listen to the voice of God and understand every day more and more how God wants to use me to do his work. I am a Prophet; he reveals to me in any way he wants to. My job is just to obey and follow the command. No two Prophets are the same; each person operates differently. I can't expect God to speak to me in the same way he does to other Prophets. Saints, what I am trying to say is that when you have a relationship with God, you will know how God speaks to you, and you will be able to function in your calling without any doubt.

6. Anger

The spirit of anger comes in most of the time when you face rejection, confusion and misunderstanding about your calling. You know you have been called in a certain field, but it seems like nobody understands you, or you don't want to accept the fact that you are called for that. When you try to say or do something as you are led by the Spirit of God, you feel you are being judged. It seems like you are not allowed to make mistakes. You have to do your job perfectly and without any error. I remember when I first started with my ministry, I used to prophesy as the word came. Back then, the wisdom of God was not so strong on me as it is now. I used to prophesy to everyone everywhere. I was not very conscious of the environment and whether the people believed me or not. I would just speak. There was even a time I told a woman, "Your husband is unfaithful and he is sleeping around." We were in a group then, and what I didn't realize then is that the woman didn't want the rest of the group to hear that, so she tried to push me away from the group to talk to me. Now, I know better. With certain prophecies, the wisdom of God needs to be applied. Well, even though she admitted what I was saying was true, she was not happy with me and the prophesy. She decided to ban me from her life.

Many times in the past, I prophesied to people about things going on in their marriages, and even though they knew it was true, they would just ban me from their lives. I used to feel lonely and bad about that. I was even afraid to keep prophesying at certain points. I got angry with myself, God and even the people I was prophesying to. I just wanted to be left alone. But it doesn't work like that. The gift and calling upon your life is irrevocable (Romans 11:29). It was given by God for life and can't be withdrawn. Even if you refuse to walk in your gift or calling, it remains forever part of you. You can run, but you can't hide from the gift or calling upon your life. You will have to pick yourself up, deal with whatever anger you are going through and get ready for the assignment, because every single day there will be a challenge that you will need to deal with.

7. Discouragement

Discouragement is also part of your shaping process. Yes, you will get discouraged over and over. People will look down on you, talk bad to you, steal your work and achievements for their own glory, reject you, try to embarrass you, lie about you, bring confusion and so much more. But you can't let discouragement stop you. King David encouraged himself in the Lord.

If you know you are called for a certain field, then call out to the one and only God that can help you. It is our Father in heaven that gave you the assignment, and he is the only one that can teach and train you in how to fulfill that assignment. He will send you help, such as destiny helpers that will come into your life to speak a word and activate and unlock all that needs to be unlocked in you. He always sends his best help at the right time and right season. Be led always by the Spirit of God, and may you encourage yourself in the Lord and not seek for people to encourage you, because most of the time they will let you down. Study the Word of God and apply it. Don't let discouragement stop you from fulfilling your divine calling.

8. Wrong doctrine

There are many different doctrines out there that can deviate you from the true word of God. But there is one book that will always tell you the truth: the Holy Bible. Before you start following people or reading all sorts of Christian books or scholarly papers, read the Bible for yourself and discover God's pattern for how you're supposed to run your ministry. Know what the Word is saying about a matter in your ministry. Don't just take a message and start running with it because this is what John Doe taught you. Confirm it with the Word of God. Find out for yourself from the Word of God if it is true.

The problem most people run into is that they hear a message, and because it sounds good, it sounds powerful, it sounds like a word many would like, they just start running with it. By the time they are questioned about it and they haven't done their homework, they get stuck. They have no proper answer or solid root to back up that word. Why? They got it from somebody and never took time to confirm it with the Word of God, so now they are stuck. If you make this mistake, people might even call you fake. You are running with something that is not biblical, and you are trying to convince yourself and others that it is biblical. Watch out for wrong doctrines!

"Now I urge you, brothers, to watch out for those who create divisions and obstacles that are contrary to the teaching you have learned. Turn away from them." (Romans 16:17)

9. Confusion

The spirit of confusion comes in sometimes, and its main goal is to destroy you. We don't serve a confusing God, but a God of order. Whatever is going wrong in your life that you know is bringing confusion, deal with it fast. Confusion brings quarrels, lies and chaos. I remember there was a time in my life when I had to deal with so many confusions – from one confusion to another. And to make my situation worse, a close friend asked me one day in anger, "So, why is it that everyone is wrong? Are you so holy that you are not making mistakes?" Coming from this person's mouth it really hurt me. It shut me down. I just stopped talking and let God fight my battle for me. I just didn't have any more strength to deal with all the confusion and misunderstanding that was going on. I just took a step back and watched how people were treating me, talking about me behind my back, laughing at me, looking down on my ministry and on me as a person. I felt very lonely then. But I decided to trust God. I just said, "God, you will not make me come this far for nothing. Make a way for me."

After a few years, God himself vindicated me. One day, God just showed up on my behalf and delivered my from every struggle. God started vindicating me publicly. I think that is when my love for God and his people got even stronger. Why? I saw Satan trying to destroy me and the work God gave me. I know he was behind the evil attacks all the time. But when God vindicated me in the way he did it. I started to get my self-confidence back, and all I could feel was love. Tears of joy were rolling from my eyes for days.

If you are dealing with this spirit of confusion, bind it and allow God to step in the boat and vindicate you. You will be able to walk on water then.

10. The seed not falling on good ground

One day a spiritual daughter called me and said, "Mama, I don't understand how come a person that is serving God for so long can still end up making wrong decisions most of the time. Shouldn't that person be wiser and know better?" I understood her question right away. I told her, "I understand your question. Let me take you to the Word of God, the Parable of the Sower." She said, "Parables again? You always speak in parables." I asked her, "Don't they come through?" She just smiled, because she is always telling me, "Mama, everything you prophesy always happens, so I need to listen when you talk or prophesy." I took her to Matthew 13 and asked her to read verses 1-23 of that chapter. Each time she read, I would try to break it down for her just to make sure she understood what she was reading. As she was reading, she said, "Wow, I never knew this." She was shocked to read that the seed which is the word of God can fall on four grounds, and that the ground on which it falls will show in the behavior of the person.

If the seed doesn't fall on good ground, it doesn't matter how much people tell you are called, you will keep on rejecting it. You just lack knowledge of the true word of God for you to grow into your calling. Unless you start meditating and studying the Bible more, the seed will never be able to fall on good ground for you to grow. Each person will have to examine themselves and find out how much of the word of God they really know. "Do I really know what it means to serve God, to be elected by God to serve in the fivefold or called by God as a businessman or woman?" That is why, before your ordination or your first step into the business field, you must have proper training and skills to operate well in your calling. Stepping into your calling doesn't just happen by night. You will have to go through some training before that oil comes upon your head.

One of my spiritual daughters was being prepared for her ordination, and I told her, "You will have to write an exam as you are being prepared for your ordination. That exam will be on paper but also physical. Because around the time of your ordination, some terrible life lessons usually come, just like what I went through with the loss of my brother one month before my ordination." She was like, "I am going through so many strange things at the moment, things I have never been through before." I said to her, "Those are all part of the practical exam. Don't fail, but come out strong."

Saints, don't let the devil or anyone else stop you from walking into your ministry when you know you are called. Take a stand and fight the battle, first spiritually in prayer and fasting, and by the time it starts manifesting physically, it becomes a small problem you can handle. Make sure you are always one step ahead of the challenge. Don't let little challenges become big battles because you fail to do what you are supposed to do. That is the time and season to be closer to God like never before. Engage yourself in a lot of prayer, fasting and mediation on the Word of God before you step into your ministry, because the challenges are going to come, and if you are not well armed with the sword, which is the Word of God, you will reject the calling.

11. Painful situations (life lessons)

Some people are constantly fighting all sorts of battles with no good knowledge of the Word of God. They start doubting God and drift away from everything that has to do with God. But that was not my case – for me, my pain drew me even closer to God.

In 2016 when I was going through some rough life lessons, I realized I would become hopeless if I didn't obey the calling and serve God faithfully. In April of that year, my young brother passed, as I explained in the previous chapter. But in that same year on May 31st, my husband and I were going to be ordained: he as an Apostle and I as a Prophet. During the months of April and May, I remember living two lives. First, I needed to mourn and be with my family; secondly, I needed to stay focused and listen to the voice of God to do his work. It felt like I had no choice and nobody to talk to about what was going on in my heart. I was like one person with two different brains: one brain processing "Why did my brother have to die like that?" and the other brain in sharp discernment and speaking to all about Jesus.

Looking back, it was a very strange period of my life. In those two months, I passed through so much pain and rejection. My family was grieving, and a lot of very painful things were said and done to each other. But there was a spirit of boldness that came upon me each time my family came nearby. One day my sweet granny was in so much pain, and I looked at her straight into the eyes and said, "Granny, God loves you, Jesus loves you." The more I kept on repeating that, the angrier she got. I even raised my voice to her, telling her, "Jesus loves you." Suddenly, she took a kettle with hot water to throw it on me. She said, "If you don't stop saying that, I will throw this hot water on you." I said to her, "Throw it, I am not afraid, but Jesus still loves you."

Right that moment, she jumped back to her senses and just pulled back, because she was standing in front of me, ready to throw hot water on me. From her face, I saw she was feeling bad about what just happened. I left and went to my mom's house. But as I was there, the Spirit of God started speaking to me. God told me, "Clearly your sweet granny didn't mean anything she said. She is just grieving. But you need to go back and apologize to her." I was like, "Apologize for what? She was the one that wanted to throw hot water on me." God said. "You raised your voice in front of your grandmother – you disrespected her." Immediately, I went back to my grandmother's house and apologized to her. I said, "Granny, I love you, and I am sorry if I hurt you." She just looked at me so sweetly, it was like the incident with the hot water had never happened.

When my grandmother was holding that kettle with hot water, ready to throw it on me, I felt a sudden growth in the Spirit I had never felt in my life. There was such a spirit of boldness that came upon me to speak to her. I remember feeling that day, right that moment, like a strong giant not afraid to die for Jesus. I felt so strong and confident that no matter what, I just had to tell her Jesus loves her. I knew then that I was not grieving, I was busy with my ministry. I needed my grandmother to see that she must keep the faith and willingness to live, because she was grieving and had started rejecting food. She was getting weaker and weaker every day, spiritually and physically. I knew I had to minister to her and let her know there is still hope for the living.

After the burial of my brother, I came home and spent time praying and fasting as I prepared for the ordination. I prepared a dance with a few Eagle sisters and went to be ordained as the Lord's vessel on the 31st of May, 2016, about a month after the death of my little brother. All that was going through my mind was "I have no choice. Serving God is not an option for me – it is a must." I couldn't look back; there was too much pain and suffering. I needed to look forward. There was something better for me ahead.

I never had the audacity to challenge God about me serving him after the death of my brother. It never came to mind. All I knew was that I had to move on with my life. My brother came to earth and left, but I am still on earth with an assignment that I must fulfill. I am using the word "must" because not for one second did I allow my painful situation to say no to my ordination. There was this full conviction in me that, yes, I was called to be a Prophet of God despite the pain I was going through.

12. Dissatisfaction, envy and jealousy

Whatever you are called for, it is God that chooses his elected ones, and when you answer to the call, you can function well in your ministry. But you need to know the requirements and expectations of each calling and stay in your lane. Don't envy another person. If you know you are called to be an Evangelist but want to operate as an Apostle or Prophet because you think those titles are much more respected, you are on the wrong track. Or if you are called to be a Pastor but you choose to become a businessman because you believe you will earn more money faster, then you will struggle, because Pastor is your calling, not businessman. But if you are called to be a businessman, be a businessman who knows the word of God: a businessman who is not money driven, a thief, a liar and corrupt but who wants to serve the needs of the people through business. You want to offer your services to a problem – to be a problem solver. Or if you are called to be a politician, you are called to make the world a better place, not to steal from the people.

My husband always tells me, "If you are called to be a Prophet, be the best Prophet you can be. Don't try to impress others by trying to operate in other callings if you know you are called for something else. There are people every year who change their office or their business; those are just confused people not hearing from God. Don't envy any ministry, just operate in the ministry you are called and carry the cross."

Not one ministry is easy. If you are called to operate in the fivefold ministry, you will need to discover your office (job description) and get the proper training in how to operate in your office from teachings, schools, trainings, church leaders, mentors and spiritual parents. I remember when I was being prepared as a Prophet, I had weekly contact with my spiritual parents. Then it was just my spiritual father, who taught me so much about my Prophetic office. But there is one thing he taught me that I will never forget. I remember when he was going through a lot of pain, sufferings and persecution, he would talk to me with all the grief in his heart, and all he could say was "Daughter, no matter what, love. Love God's people. You can't operate in the prophetic if you don't love God and his people." That stuck in my head till this day. You must do what God tells you to do even if you know the people will stone you. Be God's Prophet and not the people's Prophet." Those words taught me so much. I learned how to know when it is time to disconnect from people. When they start telling you what to prophesy (instead of you prophesying) or trying to get you to agree with them on things that are not part of the plan of God, you'd better start running very fast and not look back. Be the Lord's Prophet and not the people's Prophet.

Most of the time, you see the Apostle working together with the Prophet, and the Teacher with the Pastor, while the Evangelist is outside on the streets gathering the people to bring them to church. Each office comes with its own struggles and cross to carry. If you try to walk in an office you were not ordained by God to work in, you will have to deal with a heavy weight that you are not able to carry. God only gives what he knows you need to fulfill his given assignment and not your own heart's desires. If you are called to be a businessman, then create jobs for others with your business, work with other businesses, study the market, do research, educate yourself and make sure you catch up with the latest happenings in the market – and also learn how to be a blessing to others with your business. It is not always about the money and "if you don't pay, I can't serve you." There are some times you need to bless people with your business. Don't focus only on how to get rich fast with your business. I have news for you: most of the time, the real cash, the profit, starts flowing after two years in your business. When you have worked hard in the business for it to grow, pay your tithes, pay honest salaries to your employees and really serve the needs of the people. Serve in your ministry with excellence.

Saints, stay in your lane! Doing the job you are not called for will wear you out, and it can kill you before your time. A man of God once said, "If you die early, you will go to heaven and carry bricks because your room is not ready." Since you came early to heaven, you will have to help carry the bricks to prepare your room. Please don't be dissatisfied with your calling or envious of other callings. Enjoy the job and always give your best.

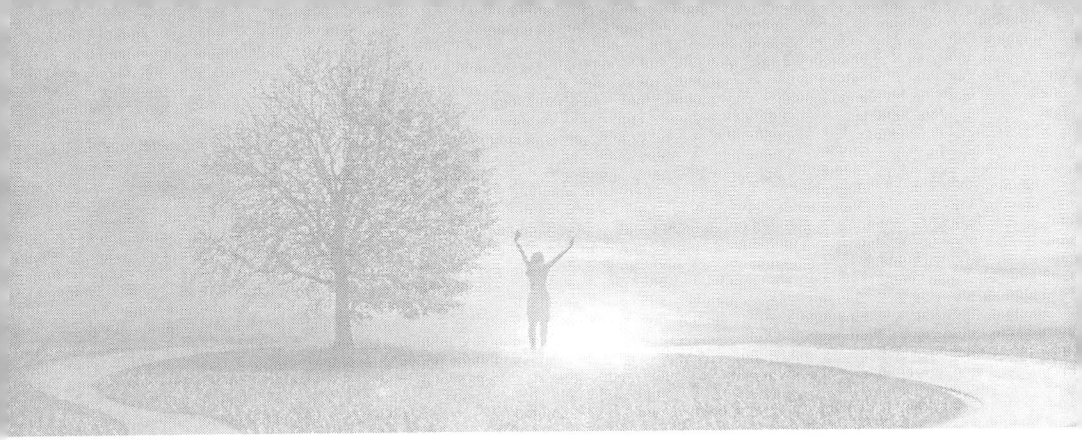

Chapter 5

The Fruits of Your Works

"If we love our Christian brothers and sisters who are believers, it proves that we have passed from death to life. But a person who has no love is still dead. Anyone who hates another brother or sister is really a murderer at heart. And you know that murderers don't have eternal life within them." (1 John 3:14-15)

What are the fruits of your works?

1. Becoming a destiny helper

You become a destiny helper when you are able to be a blessing to another, in that moment when you are able to help that person who needs a destiny helper. Moses was busy in the wilderness for years leading God's people. It was not just a few people but millions. From morning to evening, he was leading God's people. But when his father-in-law Jethro saw what he was doing, he said to Moses, "The way you are working, it will kill you." There was need for adjustment in the manner Moses was working, and Jethro came and gave advice that was able to make the job easier for Moses. Jethro explained to Moses what he could adjust to make the job easier for him and the people he was leading, and Moses was willing to follow the instructions. Jethro was, at this point, not just only his father-in-law but also his destiny helper.

2. Spiritual growth

When Prophet Elijah was about to depart, he asked Prophet Elisha, "What do you want from me?" Elisha asked for a double portion of his anointing. Elijah answered and said if Elisha is still around by the time he departs, he shall receive that double portion. Elisha was indeed around, and he received that double portion of Elijah and became a Major Prophet. He grew in his calling as he received that double portion from his master.

3. Favor, honor and respect

When the Angel of God paid Gideon a visit and said, "Mighty warrior, God is with you," Gideon had found favor with God. God had already favored him and had a plan to prosper him and his family. Gideon saw his family as the weakest in Manasseh, and himself as the least important member of his family, so he couldn't understand how he was fit for the job. But God told him, "I will be with you." Gideon eventually prospered in the assignment he was called to do by God, and from the weakest and least, he became a strong and mighty warrior and gained honor and respect from men.

Just like Gideon, Noah always found favor with God, and so too can you find favor with God. He shall then make your ways prosperous, and he shall bless you in every area. And he said in his Word that if your ways are pleasing to him, he will make even your enemy at peace with you (Proverbs 16:7).

4. Success, wealth and prosperity

Joseph started very rough with his journey. From the moment he started prophesying, he ended up in the pit, then the palace, then prison. But then it was his time of victory and prosperity, and he became the prime minister and was wealthy. Where Joseph went, God was with him and prospered him. But before the prosperity, there was a story. What will be your story before your prosperity? Get ready for your story.

5. Publicity

Jesus went about from city to city preaching the gospel in power and authority, and signs and wonders followed. When the people saw the manifestations, a large crowd believed and followed him. He became popular. But when the hour came for him to finish the job at the cross, the crowd was no longer there. Most of them abandoned him.

Publicity may come as you are fulfilling your assignment,

but you must remain focused and not deviate from your assignment. With, Jesus it was not about the large crowd that was following and making him popular. It was about that large crowd that was hungry to hear the Word and see change in their lives. He had compassion for them. Stay focused!

6. Wisdom

King Solomon was known to be the wisest man ever. No one had the kind of wisdom he had. He prayed and asked God for understanding and wisdom to rule God's people, and he got it. But Solomon disobeyed God and lost all that he had. *"Fear of the LORD is the foundation of wisdom"* (Proverbs 9:10). To be able to obtain the wisdom of God and maintain it, you must fear God. With the wisdom of God, you shall achieve great things on this journey.

I remember when God gave me the vision to do, for the first time in my life, a choreography and drama production on the story of Joseph. I started writing and doing things I had never done before. I was completely led by the Spirit of God. I spoke to everyone about what I wanted to do without even knowing if it was possible. All I knew was that God was with me, guiding me. I just followed the instruction, and in the end, it became a big success in Amsterdam with a large crowd. I was even able to write and produce my first song specially for this event. It was so nice to see the outcome of my hard labor and obedience. For many, it was their first time ever seeing something like that. I can even say the same for me. By God's grace, I was able to arrange an event I had never seen or heard before, but it became a big success with a full hall. A man of God came up to me during the program and asked me: "Prophetess, why are your programs always so different and successful?" My answer was simple: "I listen to what God tells me to do, and I just do it." He left pondering.

Be a God-fearing man or woman, obey God and walk in the wisdom of God.

7. God's protection and good health

When you obey and walk according to the will and path of the Lord, he always protects you and takes care of you. "So you shall serve the Lord your God, and He will bless your bread and your water. And I will take sickness away from the midst of you. No one shall suffer miscarriage or be barren in your land; I will fulfill the number of your days" (Exodus 23:25-26). Even when it seems like the opposite, he is there watching over you. His Word said "he will order his angels to protect you wherever you go" (Psalm 91:11). "A thousand may fall at your side, and ten thousand at your right hand; but it shall not come near you. Only with your eyes shall you look, and see the reward of the wicked" (Psalm 91:7-8). There are so many promises of his protection over your life; all you need to do is believe and see it come to pass over your life. That is the will of God for us.

Chapter 6

The Authority Given to You

"For though we walk in the flesh, we do not war according to the flesh. For the weapons of our warfare are not carnal but mighty in God for pulling down strongholds, casting down arguments and every high thing that exalts itself against the knowledge of God, bringing every thought into captivity to the obedience of Christ, and being ready to punish all disobedience when your obedience is fulfilled." (2 Corinthians 10:3-6)

This morning after my author's class, my coach spoke to me and gave some tools I needed to add to my book. It was just a confirmation. During the class, God had started speaking to me, saying that I needed to write more about my personal story in the book – to take out some of those Bible verses and write more about my own personal experiences, the life lessons I went through before I started walking in my calling. I wrote nine pages in about three hours. Heaven was just downloading and bringing back all I went through and the mistakes I made and how I learned from them. God will speak through many vessels and channels to unfold his plan. Your ears and eyes will have to have a sharp, discerning spirit. Most of the time when God speaks about a subject and your mind is not there, God will just drop it in your spirit, and it is like a book full of wisdom just opened in front of you. Walking with God, you must always be ready to listen and slow to speak.

As God was speaking through my coach, I was listening because I know it was just a confirmation. It felt like it was God himself that came down in person and spoke to me. Then I was in my 21 days of prayer and fasting. The evening before my class, I prayed and asked God to open my eyes and ears to make it all clear for me – all that I need to hear and see. That is exactly what was happening as I started writing.

After writing, I prayed for a while, then went to bed. I had a dream about being with my family in a city, and we were planning on going somewhere. As we were walking, I stopped and entered a shop with my cousin and another person. They said they were thirsty, and I decided to buy them a drink. As I entered the shop, I started talking to the owner, who seemed to be a nice man. I started talking to him about God, but then his countenance and body language changed towards me. I could see clearly that he was not interested in hearing about salvation. He even walked off and left me as I was talking to him. My cousin looked at me, laughed and said, “He is not a believer. He doesn’t want to hear anything about God.” I said, “Yes, I can see that.”

Then I remember going back outside to the rest of my family waiting for us while we entered the shop. Then one family member asked the rest of them, "Does she know where we are going?" Then she looked at me and asked me, "Do you know where we are going?" I said no. She said, "We are going to hell. There is a carnival passing by and we can't miss it. We need to make sure we are on time there." My mind was not really processing well the meaning of the word "hell." It seemed like I just wanted to hurry up to join them – I couldn't miss the carnival. So I went back into the shop, but my cousin and the other person were really delaying us. Suddenly, I realized the rest of the family had left for the carnival without me. I went looking for them. Then I saw a large line of people in front of me, and a person told me the carnival already passed and I had missed it. My family was nowhere to be found.

When I woke up in the morning, I started pondering about this dream. I spoke to my husband about it. It is when I was telling him about the dream that I realized most of my family are not saved and they are going to hell. I just rebuked that dream and covered them with the blood of Jesus. I realized more prayer is needed for them. Even though I pray every day for them, most of them are not saved. I still have to work on this assignment for my family.

A few years ago, God revealed to me, "I made you a watcher over your family," meaning praying for them constantly and making sure they know Jesus. I have been given the mandate and the authority from God to uproot, pull down and plant. I know every word that comes out of my mouth is life and power; therefore, I have learned to mind my words. What I don't want to see happen or hear, I can't speak it. And what I do want to hear and see, I speak it. I receive it as already done after declaring it. That is faith! I declared my family saved and that they will not go to hell because of their lifestyle, so I speak it in authority and back it up with constant prayer – the living word of God.

I prayed for fourteen years for my mother to accept Jesus as her Lord and Savior. Now, she is a believer of Christ and even a great support of my ministry and church. I remember there were days she would literally curse me and tell me, "Stop preaching in my head. Stop trying to control my life." There were times I would get angry, but then I realized it is not by force. I can't force Jesus on her; it must be a free will. But each time I could drop a seed of the word of God in her spirit, I would do it. I didn't give up on her. Even now, when she says or does something that seems wrong, I talk to her about it. She listens and respects me, but I had to earn that respect. How did I earn it? By my actions, conduct, character and behavior. She had to see Jesus in me before she was able to believe me.

Sometimes she will mumble and grumble, so I make sure I don't add more heat to the fire, but remain as calm as I can. Sometimes I would lose control over myself and mess things up, but then we always come back to each other in love. She is and will always be my mother. I have to respect her first if I want her to respect and believe in my Jesus. Sometimes it feels like I am the mother and she is the daughter. We talk about that and just laugh. The bottom line is, she is being saved and receiving eternal salvation staying on the right track with God. Now, my mother is my number one fan, she encourages me, supports my ministry and is always looking for a way to bless me or the ministry with whatever I need. When I am sad, I don't need to talk much; she just looks at me and says, "Sherma, you are worried, I can see it." She would say "Stop stressing" – or in Papiamento, our local language, in Curaçao, "stop di laga hende kansabu" (meaning "stop letting people worry you"). They will kill you before your time.

Because you are walking in power and authority, God can use you to speak to anybody and anything. You just need to be aware of the power you are carrying. As you speak the word of God, signs and wonders will follow as you act in authority – that authority that Jesus had when he walked here on earth. Jesus was never afraid to speak the truth. He even rebuked his family when they didn't understand his assignment. His own mother and brothers called him mad. Jesus said, "*'Who is my mother, and who are my brothers? Pointing to his disciples, he said, 'Here are my mother and my brothers. For whoever does the will of my Father in heaven is my brother and sister and mother'*" (Matthew 12:48-50). He didn't have time to think and worry whether they would still like him or if he was disrespecting his family. He was speaking the truth.

When you are speaking the truth, you can never disrespect

a person. But the problem we have in this generation is that from the moment the truth comes out, if that person looks down on you or doesn't believe in your calling, they will start insulting you to make you feel bad. They will even try to find some supporters to insult you more and make you feel like you are the worst person in the world. Don't get caught up with those deceiving tricks! Whether it is mother, father, leader or whoever, God wants you to speak to them. Speak the truth at all times. That will set you and the other person free. If they choose to believe you, praise the Lord; if they don't believe you, shake off the dust and move on. You can keep them in prayer, but don't let them discourage you or make you feel less. You have been given power and authority – walk in it at all times!

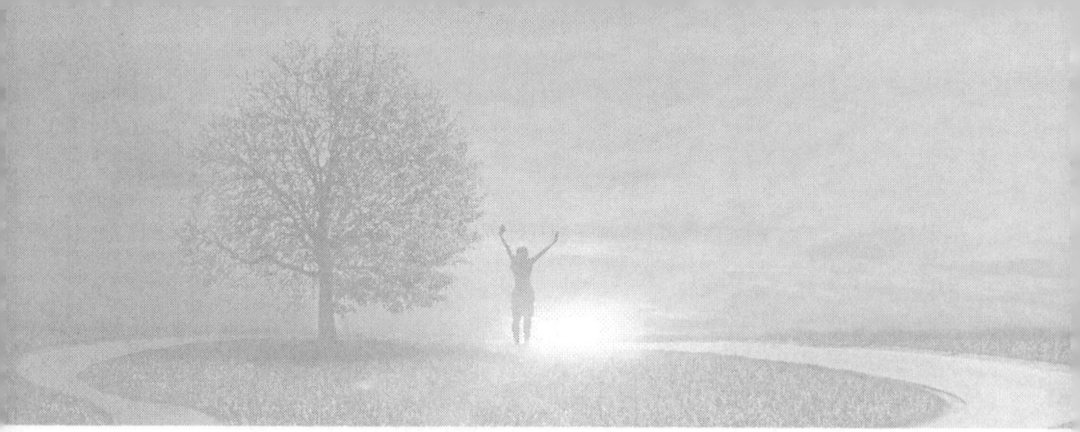

Chapter 7

Bruised but Not Broken to Answer the Call

"I can do all things through Christ who strengthens me." (Philippians 4:13)

"Fear not, for I am with you; be not dismayed, for I am your God. I will strengthen you, yes, I will help you, I will uphold you with My righteous right hand." (Isaiah 41:10)

"The Lord is my strength and song, and He has become my salvation; He is my God, and I will praise Him; my father's God, and I will exalt Him." (Exodus 15:2)

The path to answering to God's call may have not been easy. Maybe you have been bruised many times, but that shouldn't stop you from answering to the call.

If you can just see it as an honor to be chosen by God for the assignment, it can make your walk with God easier.

Going through the pain and struggles is all part of the assignment to make you stronger and wiser. If you can just hold on and press on, you will make it.

If you can just understand and be encouraged in the Lord, then the bruises will come, but they will not last forever. The brokenness is meant to shape and correct you.

If you can just see that Jesus is in the boat with you, and that he wants you to trust him and step out of the boat just like Apostle Peter did, you will make it.

If you can just rely on him and trust not on your own understanding, you will make it.

If you allow the Holy Spirit to guide you and your destiny helpers to help you, you will make it.

If you stop walking behind God and start walking side by side or in front of God, just like Abraham did, you will make it.

If you allow yourself to grow from your mistakes and don't see yourself as "once a failure, forever a failure," you will make it.

If you can move from faith to trust you will make it. Trust in God!

Chapter 8

Prayer for You to Discover and Grow into Your Calling

Lord Jesus, I thank you for the precious gift of life

I thank you for your blood that was shed for us

I thank you for making us the apple of your eye

I thank you for calling us your very own, your chosen people, a royal priesthood

Lord, we were the least of all, but you called us to be your very own.

Today I pray the name of Jesus Christ, and I bind every Sanballat and Tobiah spirit that is trying to confuse or stop your people from answering to your call. I bind every Jezebel spirit that is trying to silence your people and kill the vision. I declare that every person still believing in you will discover their calling and assignment here on earth – you shall make a way for them. To every spiritual blindness, dumbness or deafness, I say be open in Jesus' name. Lord, open their spiritual eyes and ears and sharpen the spirit of discernment of your people to be sensitive to your voice. Lord, I pray that they may hear you and harken unto your voice.

May they no longer be discouraged, distracted or in doubt that they will hear you and answer to the call.

Lord, I thank you for everyone operating in their calling. I ask for more of your grace and protection over them.

Lord, I thank you for the destiny helpers that will help your people fulfill their God-given assignment here on earth.

Lord, I thank you for the open doors that your people will step in as they are led by the Holy Spirit. And every wrong door, I declare them shut.

Lord, I declare that your people shall rule and reign and become great, leaving a legacy behind for their children and grandchildren.

Lord, I declare this book a blessing unto all who read it. They shall have full understanding of their calling and how to go about it to fulfill their colorful destiny.

This is declared in Jesus' name. Amen.

Another title by
Sherma Oriakhi-Merselina

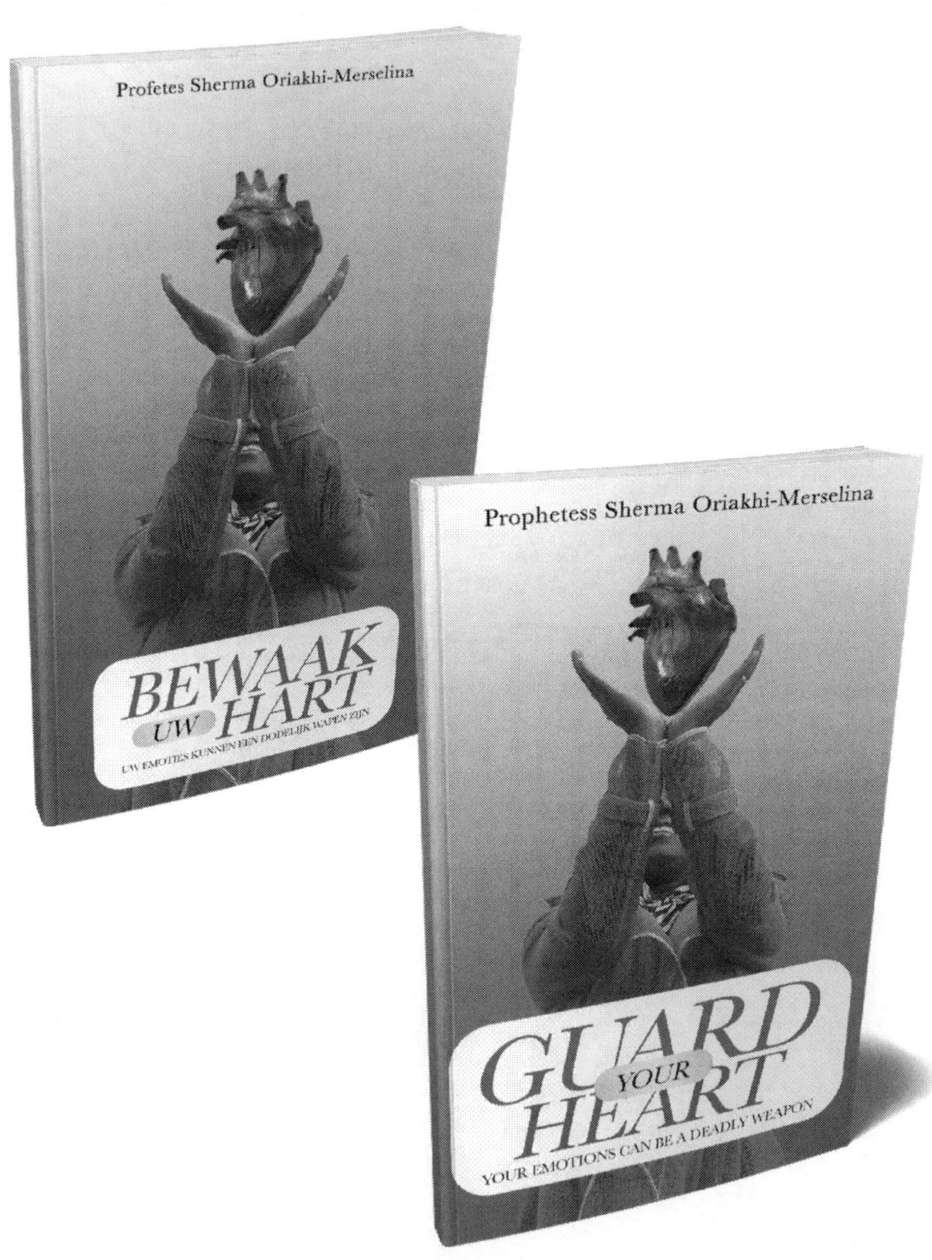

Made in the USA
Columbia, SC
29 April 2025